BREAKING
—— OUT OF ——
BURNOUT

How to Overcome
Mid-Career Burnout and
Come Back Stronger

REX BAKER

© 2019 Rex Baker Enterprises

Rex Baker

All rights reserved, including the right of reproduction in whole or in part in any form whatsoever, whether printed, audio, electronic or digital.

Rex can be contacted at rex@rexbaker.net
Visit his website at www.rexbaker.net
Subscribe to his Youtube channel, "The Attic Library", to receive Rex's weekly book reviews.

Book design by Old Mate Media
Published by Rex Baker Enterprises

Printed by KDP Paperback

First Edition

ISBN   978-1-7335308-0-4 Print
           978-1-7335308-1-1 Digital

Special Thanks

I dedicate this book to my family. First, to my wife Carol, who believed in me when this book was a mere spark in my imagination. Next, to my daughters, Hillary and Rachel, who will always be "Daddy's little girls."

I would not have written this book without my Mother, who taught me her love of reading and books. Finally, I dedicate this book to my older special needs brother Perry, who fought the good fight against cancer, telling me right up until the end, "I'm getting better." Today, Perry is in a better place, free of cancer and physical limitations.

It is with Perry's eternally optimistic spirit that I wish you, the reader of this book, a determined victory in breaking out of burnout.

Introduction

Career job burnout is at epidemic levels today, leaving countless people questioning their choice of profession or point in life. If you are burned out, you may wonder if you'll ever be happy again. Burnout leaves you emotionally drained and devoid of contentment in one of our most important facets of life, our jobs.

You may deal with people all day long who don't appreciate your hard work. Perhaps you have a supervisor who always demands more but never utters a simple "thank you." Your customers or clients complain or berate you for not working faster, yet the company won't hire more help.

You work all day, only to rush from work to pick up the kids, start dinner, wash clothes and help with homework and wake up the next day to start the rat race all over again. It wasn't supposed to be this way.

Fortunately, there is hope. In this book, we will lay out practical ways to rejuvenate your life and bring purpose to your step. These proven and tested methods will put you back where you belong, *in control of your life.*

I overcame burnout in my own career and know the power of the processes laid out in these pages. I have also implemented morale-boosting practices with the employees in my workplace. I've done the hard work of putting together this program because I want you to achieve victory over burnout and forge a new path in your life.

If you apply the teachings in this book, you will regain a passion for your life and career. You will learn how to get the right people in your life to help you grow, *and how to put the wrong people who are holding you back on the shelf.* You will become adept at listening to the right voices and tuning out the critics and naysayers.

If you do the hard work of applying the principles put forth in this book, you will break out of burnout and bounce back stronger than before. These principles are so powerful they can't help but transform your life if you work them.

You have an enemy!! That enemy is procrastination, the little voice in your head that says you'll do it tomorrow, next week, next month. However, tomorrow never comes. You only have "today", so make it count and get started working your *Breaking Out of Burnout* program right now.

Where to start? Simple. ***You start by reading this book.*** Set a goal of finishing the book because finishing what you start is a hallmark principle of overcoming burnout. Therefore, start your *Breaking Out of Burnout* program and begin breaking out of your own personal burnout by reading this book to completion. I am truly excited for the journey you are about to begin!

Author's Warning: If properly applied, the disciplines in this book can transform your life. However, be aware this book is not for everybody.

WARNING!
DO NOT READ THIS BOOK IF:

- You are looking for a quick fix.
- You are not willing to take risks.
- You don't want to do the work of investing in yourself.
- You're content being a conformist who follows the crowd.
- You aren't comfortable being challenged.

ONLY READ THIS BOOK IF:

- You're willing to do the work to regain your passion and drive.
- You have an unfulfilled life dream.
- You know deep inside you're not pursuing your dream.
- You want to create a legacy, and leave this world better than you found it.
- You welcome the challenge of a lifetime.

When you complete the book, please leave an honest review on Amazon!

If you are burned out and seek to regain control of your life, download my free resource and start the journey of rebuilding your life today.

4 Steps to Taking Back Your Life by Taking Back Your Day

https://rexbaker.ck.page/95c215070d

Contents

Part 1 **The Problem** 1
1. My Story 3
2. What is Burnout 9
3. Workplace Burnout 13
4. What Type of Person Are You? 19
5. It's Your Problem--Own It! 29
6. Hope Stealers 37

Part 2 **The Great Awakening** 45
7. No Excuses 47
8. Where to Start 53
9. Listening to the Right Message 63
10. Prepare for the Backlash 73
11. Taking Action 81
12. Making the Right Friends 89
13. The Books You Read 97
14. Breakout Habits 105
15. Action Plan 113
16. Conclusion 117

PART 1

THE PROBLEM

CHAPTER 1
MY STORY

On Christmas morning 1997, I wished the viewers of our 6:00 a.m. newscast a Merry Christmas from my television anchor desk. Meanwhile, my two little daughters awakened to Santa's wondrous delights. I missed that Christmas morning with my daughters, never to be relived again.

That morning drove the nail in the coffin of putting a job before my family. Never again would I miss a Christmas morning with my children so a corporation could make money. Three months later, I walked out of the world of television news with my head held high.

I didn't know what to call it back then, but after 15 years in the television news business, I had burned out. A profession that initially offered high job satisfaction and the opportunity to make a positive difference turned into a meat-grinder that stressed quantity over quality.

Our modern society is tailored for burnout. People working in high-stress jobs, who want to make a difference, set themselves up as prime candidates for burnout. Folks across the professional spectrum are running on empty hoping to make it to the weekend, so they can get a quick refuel before Monday morning comes calling. It often comes as a shock when what was once considered a dream job turns into a nightmare.

As a reporter, I covered presidential visits, interviewed national political leaders, and kept my pulse on the local political scene. I loved my job and took pride in the profession. Sure, we griped privately about the low pay and the heavy workload, but youthful energy and idealism overrode the downside. However, as the years ticked by, I began to privately ask myself, "Is this what I want to do the rest of my life?"

About a year earlier, I had begun volunteering at a local homeless shelter. I felt drawn to this strange, foreign work that existed unseen under society's nose. Monday-night chapel became my time to become friends with the drug addicts, released felons, and alcoholics that filled the rosters of the shelter's rehabilitation program.

Sammie and Robert stood out among the "program guys," and the three of us developed a bond that continues today. While talking to them one night, it dawned on me that if I followed this passion, it would mean putting down the microphones and cameras and starting over in a new line of work.

After a period of soul searching and prayer, I walked away from a television news career and entered the homeless ministry in March 1998. I remain friends with many I knew in the news business and respect those who are still working to report the news. However, I never missed another Christmas morning with my children. I was there for their school plays, recitals, and marching band competitions. I've got some regrets, but missing my kids growing up is not one of them.

Tip: *Changing jobs is not always the right answer to burnout. But if you're going to leave your job, make sure you've got another opportunity in the wings. Leave on your terms, and don't burn bridges.*

In 2003, I became the Executive Director of Gateway Rescue Mission. The challenges of running a homeless shelter jumped on my back the first day. We had more bills than money to pay them, but managed to get through the next several years. I poured my soul into taking this small organization to the proverbial next level.

Leading an organization tasked with helping dysfunctional people lit my fire and doused any thought of burnout. Helping people brought satisfaction that money couldn't buy. Short-term struggles could be justified because of the noble work of helping the homeless. We launched a fundraising program in 2007 that helped pay the bills and upgraded old facilities as money allowed. Yet, the improvements didn't come quickly or easily.

As Executive Director, I had responsibility for every part of the organization. My job encompassed fundraising, writing newsletters, dealing with employee conflict, handling insurance reports, fielding complaints, and annual reports, ad nauseam. The demands of the job required spending large amounts of time and energy doing things I hated. I was drawn to this work out of a desire to help people, not to spend countless hours writing employee policy manuals.

Part of being an adult means learning to do the things you don't like. So, I sucked it up. I read books on employee management and how to become better organized, how to become the leader your organization needs, and how to raise a gazillion dollars for your non-profit, and how to be, essentially, "perfect."

Somewhere along the line, it dawned on me that running a homeless shelter was tougher than I thought it would be. I had attended Seminary, but didn't take the first class on basic management or leadership. We learned Greek and Hebrew, systematic theology, and church history but nothing on how to deal with a disagreeable employee.

I don't know when I first heard it, that voice deep inside that says, "I don't want to do this anymore." Maybe it was when I had to personally fire an employee and friend for stealing or deal with that bogus insurance claim or the late-night work-related email that said, "You haven't responded to my email. I need you to look into this." Maybe it was being asked once again by an employee to drop what I'm doing and help them with what they're doing. Though I ignored this voice, it kept returning. By 2014, I knew something had to give. My negative emotions pointed to burnout. I took vacations, read inspirational books, went off for a few days on a personal retreat, yet the voice wouldn't shut up. I began to question my calling. I thought about returning to news reporting. God seemed strangely silent. The only thing that kept me from walking out the door for some other pasture was knowing that I had been Divinely called to this position, and the call had not been rescinded.

However, I also knew that if something didn't change, a crash was inevitable. Unlike my days in the news business, this burnout was much more intense and harder to extinguish. No longer could I just pray about it for a few weeks and have God parachute a miraculous answer into my lap. I had a family, kids in college and a mortgage. This time around, no second job appeared on the horizon.

Tip: Somebody has to do the job that nobody likes. This means that on any job, you will have to perform certain duties you don't like. Just make sure that you pay adequate attention to the vital things that only you can do rather than being pulled under by the tyranny of the urgent.

Burnout sapped my energy. Life seemed to go by in slow motion, with a proverbial ball and chain psychologically attached each day. I felt stuck in career mediocrity while watching friends build successful businesses. I felt powerless to change, yet knew the cost of not changing would enact a toll fatal to my career and purpose in life.

But one day I took one step. That one step started a journey that led to rediscovering my passion and opening up a new way of thinking and doing. That journey will continue throughout life, but I will never go back to being burned out again. While a degree of burnout may be inevitable, how we respond is not. Nothing guarantees that "it's all going to be alright." We have to take action to change the course.

Through experience, I learned that recovery from burnout is possible but not automatic. Some people stall out in life but then fight like crazy to breakout of burnout. Others bog down in life and stay stuck, or, worse yet, never get going. While each of us is unique, most people belong to a general type that determines the likelihood of overcoming burnout. Examining and knowing which type of person you are, plays a vital role in breaking out of burnout.

CHAPTER 2
WHAT IS BURNOUT

In the mid 20th Century, the term burnout often referred to rocket engines that had run out of fuel and crashed. By the 1970s, researchers were applying the term to people who had run out of fuel in their career. Psychologist Herbert Freudenberger coined the term "burnout" when working with volunteer addiction counselors at drug treatment centers. More on that later. Merriam-Webster Dictionary defines burnout as "exhaustion of physical or emotional strength or motivation usually as a result of prolonged stress or frustration."

Burnout sneaks up on you. At first, you may experience frustration from stress that doesn't go away. The stress often comes from unresolved job pressures, such as chronic overwork. Job duties increase and job satisfaction decreases. This stress can feel like a low to medium grade depression and may lead to a pessimistic view of life. Yet, since the cause is situational rather than clinical, medication is not an effective cure.

The stressor can also be a job plus kids or serving as a caregiver to a sick or elderly family member. Rather than go away, these scenarios rear their ugly heads day after day. You may complain about the situation at first without realizing the danger of burning out.

We all face stress in life. A student may complain of burnout from exams and research papers. This stress ends upon graduation. As long as you can see light at the end of the tunnel, the burnout isn't fatal.

We are concerned primarily with pervasive, long-term career burnout. In early stages, burnout may be experienced as a bad week or month. A vacation, a quick getaway and you'll be fine. However, long-term burnout doesn't end with a few days off.

When the alarm buzzes in the morning, you do not want to get up. You feel lethargic and may quit caring about your job. You are physically and emotionally exhausted. You may resent your employer or the people you once desired to help. You may even question your choice of profession.

People in early burnout often try to work their way out of it. They realize something isn't right and work harder to regain their former energy and passion. However, instead of renewing their energy, the burnout deepens and leads to lethargy. An individual who has never experienced depression may not want to get out of bed and face the day due to burnout. It's common for people who have burned out to wonder whether to remain in the profession they once found fulfilling.

Many people in burnout continue doing their jobs, sometimes even admirably. However, they don't perform at their full capacity. Even when they appear to be functioning to those around them, their work performance suffers because they quietly decide to not work to their full potential or simply cannot due to burnout.

The burnout mindset is epidemic in government jobs, where the lure of government retirement benefits keep many people trapped in jobs long after they've burned out. These employees would leave their job for the private sector in a heartbeat if not for the fact that they can retire with a defined benefit in a few years. That same worker in the private sector could consider switching jobs.

Burnout often leads to physical exhaustion. The body may translate burnout related stress into physical illness. Headaches, ulcers, body pain, digestive disorders, weakened immune systems, and other physical ailments are often a direct result of stress-related burnout.

As burnout intensifies, some people turn to increased alcohol or prescription drug use. A burned-out employee may not have the authority to change an adverse work situation. However, that same employee can make the choice to have a couple of drinks and a nerve pill at night.

Some people in burnout begin practicing risky behavior that defies their profession. A burned-out pastor may have an affair or a police officer might extort money from drug dealers. This does not mean that people who engage in immoral or illegal behavior should use burnout as an excuse. It simply means that in certain situations, burnout can lead to risky behavior that runs opposite of a profession's expected norms.

To compound the problem, many people in helping professions have difficulty asking for help. Teachers, doctors, police officers, counselors, non-profit executives, and clergy represent professions where the practitioner is expected to have the answers for other people's problems. Such professionals often have trouble asking for help because they see themselves as the person who helps others.

In working among the homeless and addicted, I have observed that burnout causes a dichotomy. People begin a career in the helping professions with a passion to see lives changed. However, the sheer enormity of the human need often overwhelms helping organizations and their employees. The case manager with a never-ending list of needy clients, the pharmacist standing on her feet all day serving lines of impatient customers, and the teacher with an overcrowded classroom of noisy kids all enter their professions with an idealistic view of helping others.

Yet, when burnout strikes after constant stress, the case manager, the pharmacist, and the teacher may withdraw and become distant from the very people they initially wanted to help. The counselor begins to view the drug-addicted clients as hopeless losers. The pharmacist views grumpy customers as an interruption or a teacher sees students as lazy and unwilling to learn. The burned-out police officer views everyone walking the streets as a criminal and the pastor views parishioners as lazy sinners unwilling to change.

Thus, a result of burnout is often cynical resentment toward those you are charged with helping. As the burnout intensifies, burned-out people experience a decrease in the satisfaction of performing their roles. In turn, they decrease personal investment in their job. This leads to lower performance rates, which causes a negative self-image.

Burned-out people know they are underperforming on the job and often blame themselves. If they only worked harder or smarter they wouldn't be having this problem. They often compare themselves to friends or colleagues who appear to be successful and think "if I were smart or charming or well-connected like so-and-so," things would be better. But things aren't better so they blame themselves.

Blaming yourself for burnout is not synonymous with guilt. Burned-out people are more likely to feel anger than guilt. Anger at being unappreciated, overworked, used by both employer and customers. A burned-out school teacher in an overcrowded classroom is more likely to feel anger toward school administrators or parents than personal guilt for underperforming students.

Disillusionment is burnout's twin sibling. You'll rarely find someone in chronic burnout mode who is not also disillusioned. The position in life they sought and obtained has not brought satisfaction. Rather, it has brought exhaustion and disillusionment.

CHAPTER 3
WORKPLACE BURNOUT

I once met a television news reporter working a story. She lugged around a camera and tripod in what we called a "one-man-band" scenario back in my days as a reporter. When assigned one-man-band duty, it meant you are both the reporter and the photographer. Despite the casual reputation as a glamour job, journalism boasts a high burnout rate. Hard working conditions combined with low pay creates a scenario where many a starry-eyed cub reporter winds up leaving the business for another career by their mid-30s.

Just how did we get in this job-burnout situation? One hundred years ago, most Americans worked on the farm. People lived their entire lives in the same area. Communicable diseases, world wars, and economic depression made a career one part of a bigger life picture often centered around survival. After World War II, nations set about the task of building a modern world.

Idealism set in, as children of the Great Depression and World War II dreamed of a better life and therefore went to college or trade school, often the first in their family to do so. Baby boomers ushered in a new era of higher career expectations. As their parents had moved from the farm to the factory, boomers moved from the factory to the office, boardroom, or executive suite.

The Depression, World War II era also saw changes in the helping professions. After World War I, a small number of people entered human services work. As the Great Depression gave rise to institutional metropolitan poverty, these workers entered the fight against social ills like hunger and alcoholism. They operated in small organizations with almost complete autonomy to work as and with whom they wished. Organizations like Alcoholics Anonymous started in Dr. Bob Smith's house with a missionary zeal to reform alcoholics one person at a time.

Others opened homeless shelters, orphanages, and schools to deal with the social issues of the day, often operated on a small and personal basis. Charity was given to those willing to work for change or those unable to help themselves. However, it was not doled out indiscriminately to everyone. Ministers, doctors, charity workers, social workers, teachers, and nurses worked with their clientele on a first-name basis. They saw their work as a calling, but not as a pathway to career satisfaction or financial success.

These autonomous organizations were scattered, varied and not highly regulated. Society primarily held people responsible for their own actions and did not transfer responsibility for their success or lack thereof onto their teachers or ministers. The relationship between doctor and patient was local and personal.

By the 1970s, the landscape had shifted. Those autonomous organizations had grown, as had the government bureaucracy to oversee them. Today, if you run a bait shop that sells crickets, minnows, and worms you have to answer to the FBCMW (Federal Bureau of Crickets, Minnows and Worms). Today's organization has to answer to multiple federal, state, and local jurisdictions. Long gone are the days of the local doctor trading services for chickens and eggs. Today's medical personnel spend more time meeting bureaucratic regulations than they do in one-on-one patient care.

The same goes for those in education, non-profits, and practically any other professional service provider arena. The church remains the sole entity that hasn't come under total government oversight and that development is likely only a matter of time.

Throw into the mix the fact that many entering the workplace today carry idealistic goals of career satisfaction and financial success. People in today's world expect a higher level of success from life. They've been programmed to achieve beyond what their parents achieved. When that doesn't happen, burnout can take place.

Also, instead of holding individuals responsible for their actions, society increasingly holds the helping professional responsible. The question becomes, "Sire Addiction Counselor, what is your success rate?" "Madam School Principal, what is the average test score of your students?" Many helping professionals internalize these expectations and indeed expect it of themselves.

When the success of the client becomes the responsibility of the professional, even if only by perception, then the professional wears the failure of the client on his or her soul. When that failure is multiplied many times over on a consistent basis, the worker is a prime candidate for burnout. This same scenario plays out daily in places like health clinics, schools, counseling offices, and mental health centers.

Many who fall into the pit of burnout started with high hopes of a brilliant career, only to see those hopes devolve into exhaustion and hopelessness. If this is you, and even if the causes of your burnout are due to circumstances beyond your control, the cure is not beyond your control.

You didn't burn out overnight. Chronic burnout among

professionals is caused by a combination of performing tasks that you either don't enjoy or don't perform well. You're like the old guy in the doughnut commercial some years ago, "time to make the doughnuts." You started with a dream of working to make a difference, but the job has devolved into the tyranny of the mundane where you feel trapped making nothing but doughnuts.

You had visions of cooking delicious steaks and whipping up exotic recipes. Sure, someone else might be happy with your daily production of sugar, calorie-laden pastries. However, you wanted more out of life than doughnuts. The daily grind of performing work you don't like combined with the unfulfilled dreams of not being allowed to do the work you like over a long period of time creates burnout.

Whether to Change Jobs

If you're burned out, when is it appropriate to look for another job? Well, it depends. As a disclaimer, *it is not within the scope of this book to determine whether you should look for employment elsewhere.* That is your prerogative as the reader. Only you can determine if a career change should be pursued.

While you may feel trapped in the job from hell, a job change is not always the smartest or best option. Other factors, such as a period of life or family pressures, may factor into your situation. Even if you work for a proverbial Vlad the Impaler, Vlad could be one more tirade away from getting his own pink slip. If your supervisor is a stinker, the weeks can seem like years. However, bad bosses often get fired, and you might quit one week before a better boss gets hired.

Tip: *Wherever you go, there you are.*

The root causes of burnout are often within us. We're burned out because we allowed ourselves to get in that situation. While it's easy to blame our employers, the scope of this book is providing practical ways to overcome burnout by changing yourself. You cannot change your supervisor. You cannot change the organization for which you work unless you are the executive or are a high-ranking supervisor. You can change yourself. Our subject in this book is about dealing with burnout rather than bad bosses.

I've been through a career change. However, my primary experience with overcoming burnout and coming back stronger took place within the context of my current employment and did not necessitate a career change. For that, I am thankful because jumping ship would have short-circuited the process that led to greater victory.

No job is perfect. While burnout can and often does lead to a career change, such a change will not make you a better person, employee, spouse, or parent. Burnout is our emotional system's way of telling us something is wrong. If that something is a dead-end job with no hope for improvement, a change may be in order. If Vlad the Impaler owns the company, consider a change. Life is too short to waste the next decade working for a jackass.

However, the focus of this book is on things within your control to improve. Whether you stay in your current position or switch careers, putting certain practices in place will ensure a better state of mind and quality of life. You don't have to let anyone else dictate your happiness.

It's good to understand some background on how we went from an agrarian society to our modern rat-racing, keep up with the Joneses world. It's "great" to face the fact that some people work for a corporation that puts the bottom line before employee satisfaction. It's certainly obvious that many people work in bureaucratic settings that drive them to seek counseling from the burned-out counselor. However, understanding accomplishes nothing unless accompanied by action.

I once had a friend who loved to complain about his life. Yet, when you pointed out a sensible explanation to a problem, he would immediately fire back with why he couldn't implement the solution. He always had to be right, and as far as I know, he still has every single problem he loved to complain about.

If you seek more information on burnout, other books are available. You can read books all day long and still be stuck. Or you can start working a program and breaking out of burnout. I've learned one fact from experience. If you start working a program to overcome burnout, you will ultimately outgrow burnout by becoming a stronger person. Do not be defined by the problem. Be defined by the solution.

The decision whether to break out of burnout is entirely yours. The power to do so lies within you. President Teddy Roosevelt said, *"it is hard to fail, but it is worse never to have tried to succeed."* I cannot predict the outcome of your journey out of burnout, but I challenge you to be among those who try to succeed, if for no other reason than to avoid the terrible regret of having never tried.

CHAPTER FOUR

WHAT TYPE OF PERSON ARE YOU

An old saying goes that *there are three types of people: Those who make it happen, those who watch it happen, and those who wonder what happened.* In this chapter, we will explore these three types and how our mindset influences our ability to overcome burnout. While anyone can burn out, one of these groups is more vulnerable to burnout. More on that later.

Burnout doesn't happen overnight. It can be like termites, eating away at the structure of your home. By the time you discover them, the damage is already underway. If the damage goes undetected too long, you face a major rehabilitation process.

Are you burned out in an important aspect of your life? Job, career, family? The first step toward getting on the right track is discovering the termites. Then you can say, "I have a problem and I know what to call it." Give that sucker a name. Its name is burnout, and it is your enemy.

Our modern concept of burnout is a relatively new phenomenon. Psychologist Herbert Freudenberger published a study in 1980 on burnout, linking it to job stress among volunteers working with drug addicts in free clinics.

Freudenberger defined burnout as a "state of mental and physical exhaustion caused by one's professional life." Research also shows that young people tend to burn out more than older adults. Yet, this finding begs a closer look.

Burnout can be short-term or long-term. Young people coming out of college often lack the maturity or boundaries between their job and personal lives. They throw themselves into a new career with reckless abandon, which leads to burnout. This "short-term" burnout can be readily treated by changing jobs, changing shifts, or maybe even taking a brief vacation.

However, middle-aged adults often get blindsided by "long-term" burnout. This more insidious form of burnout is a different monster. It won't be tamed by a week at the beach or a cruise. Burnout will only be waiting upon your return.

I'm a baby boomer, born in the early 1960s. As a teenager in the 1970s, nobody talked about burnout. Our grandparents farmed the land. Our parents worked in the factories. The majority of people lived in rural areas, with peas to pick and big lawns to mow. Mother may have attended college, or Dad went to trade school or the military. But they stayed near home. The job was one part of a rich community network that included friends, relatives, church activities, and lots of time spent outdoors doing physical labor. We ate vegetables from our own garden and went fishing if we wanted seafood.

Then we grew up and moved to the city. No more hoeing peas and cutting okra. We replaced the country yard that took three hours to mow with a small lawn that could be cut in 45 minutes. We went to Kroger for vegetables and Red Lobster for seafood. We traded the job at the factory for a promising career in the city. Instead of sending our kids out to play all day, we packed them off to daycare, while listening to the mantra from radio talk show experts on how to be the perfect parent, employee, or supervisor.

This change in focus from a self-sustaining life to one measured by elusive societal standards came at a price. The city life and career shift brought increased expectations of success. Small town life meant that activities were structured around relationships. However, in modern society activity reigns supreme. Relationships exist but often play second fiddle to the daily tyranny of activities.

When you graduate from college, you get the job, get the spouse, have some kids, buy a house. During the child-rearing years, it's all about getting junior to T-ball or soccer practice. Then comes high school football, band, cheerleading, or whatever activities your children embrace. Rather than families entwining activities through relationships, activities now often trump relationships.

Then the kids move out, go to college, and suddenly it's an EMPTY NEST. Along the way and without noticing it, *your focus shifted to working on others and you stopped working on yourself.* This is a recipe for burnout. If this is you, take a number and join an already packed crowd. When you wake up one day and wonder, "what in the name of Jethro am I going to do with the rest of my life," don't beat yourself up. You didn't do anything wrong. It's just time for an overhaul. It will take some time, effort, and maybe even cost some money. But this overhaul could give you another 100,000 miles of productive life.

If you suffer from burnout, hope exists! Here's the good news. While you can't recover from long-term burnout overnight, you can *start the journey toward recovery in one day.* As an old boss of mine used to say, "here's what you need to do." First, determine whether you are dealing with short-term or long-term burnout. Both are symptoms of the same problem, but one is more advanced than the other. Short-term burnout will lead to long-term burnout if not addressed.

Understand this. You can deal with burnout now, or deal with it later, but you will deal with it. If you are proactive and take the proper measures now, you can rebound to a stronger, more productive life. If you ignore it, you will ultimately be sidelined with a crash in your career or family life and possibly your health. At best, you will be resigned to a living a dreary, unfulfilled life.

Your life is like a vehicle engine. Let's say you are headed on vacation, and start with a full tank of gas. You want to reach your destination as quickly as possible, so you ignore the billboards advertising the next filling station. Your fuel gauge drops below half full, but you keep going. Got to get there quick! Finally, the fuel light comes on, and the little dinging sound indicates you are critically low on fuel. Yet, you figure you can make it to the next exit. Suddenly, the engine begins to sputter, and you wind up in a dead stop along the interstate.

This is short-term burnout. You call an emergency service, and eventually, someone shows up with a gas can. Or perhaps they tow you ten miles ahead to the nearest convenience station. The shutdown costs you a few bucks, and you wind up spending more time dealing with the emergency than it would have taken to refuel when the gauge dropped below half full. This type of burnout is an inconvenience, but, with a bit of attention, you're soon back up and going.

Now take that same vehicle. You ignore the instructions to change the oil every 3,000 miles or every three months. You gas up every week, blissfully unaware of what's going on under the hood. One day you notice a bit of smoke coming out the exhaust pipe. You ignore this too, hoping it will go away. Then one day you strike out on a long trip, and a strange sound starts coming from the engine. Dark smoke billows out the exhaust pipe. The engine seizes up, shuts down, and you find yourself on the side of the road again.

This time, a refill won't cut it. You need an engine overhaul, which is much more expensive in time and money. In reality, no engine lasts forever. Sooner or later you have to perform rather expensive maintenance on your engine. Valves need replacing. Hoses and belts have to be changed. Parts wear out.

It's the same with our human body. Over time, we have to perform not only routine maintenance, but also more expensive maintenance to ensure we stay healthy. If you find yourself in long-term burnout, it's time for an overhaul.

Let's put it another way. You go to the doctor with chest pains and shortness of breath. The doctor says if you want to live, you've got to replace the burgers and fries with salads and greens. You've also got to lose 50 pounds. You go home that night, step on the scales, and read the sad numbers. Before going to sleep, you pray and ask God to help you lose 50 pounds in short order.

The next morning you wake up and step on the scales. Guess how much you are going to weigh? THE SAME AS YOU DID THE NIGHT BEFORE. You can pray till the cows come home, but you've still got to do the hard work of diet and exercise to shed the pounds and get in shape. Yes, you should pray and ask for discipline to stick with the health plan, for your doctor to apply wisdom for your care, and for supportive friends to encourage your new lifestyle. But nobody is going to get on that treadmill for you. God simply will not do for us what He expects us to do for ourselves.

It's the same with burnout. You can pray for direction, see a shrink, or watch a motivational video. But nothing will happen until you start doing the work. Sadly, not everybody does. Studies show that 83% of people do not successfully keep their New Year's resolutions. Let's go deeper now with our old saying.

There are three types of people:
Those who make it happen
Those who watch it happen
Those who wonder what happened

Think about it this way. The big game is this weekend. Two rivalry teams are playing for bragging rights. Yet, a considerable number of people will be unaware that thousands of fans are gathering just blocks away. They don't have a clue that two teams are squaring off for all the marbles. These people are apathetic. Total confusion reigns in their mind when they wander downtown and see all the traffic. ***They wonder what happened.***

Another group of folks knows exactly what is happening. But they don't want to bother with the traffic, stadium food, or getting up early to attend the game. So, they watch it on television. They root for their team from the comfort of their den and large screen television. They are interested but uninvested. ***They watch it happen.***

Then there's a third group. These folks get up early or perhaps come in the day before the game. They rent hotel rooms and tailgate. They arrive hours before the big game to get a decent parking spot. They scream, yell, and stomp the stadium seats in support of their team. On the field are the players and coaches. Together, the players, coaches, and fans converge to create a frenzied atmosphere where the game actually takes place. They have skin in the game. They are invested. ***They make it happen.***

When burnout sets in, it's easy to become apathetic. You quit caring about what happens around you. The melancholy sets in like a cloudy day. You can sense light outside but can't see the sunshine. Nothing gets created from this view of life. People who wonder what happened just get by. They may sense something is going on near them, but lack the gumption to go find out, much less take place in the activity.

Tip: People who wonder what happened don't often burn out because they are content just getting by.

The middle group is where so many people fall. They know what's happening, but ride the pine watching it all unfold. They play life safe and don't take risks. They watch it happen but don't make it happen. If not corrected, people in this group often face the end of life with regrets for never having truly attempted to fulfill their dreams. They settle for the momentary comfort of mediocrity rather than attempting the bold, exhilarating feat of doing something that really matters. And when life is at its end, and they no longer have the health, resources, or energy to live their dream, they face the agony of regret over never having gone for the gold. They watched life on television rather than making life happen in person.

Tip: Many people in long-term burnout fit this group. They have enough wits about them to know this is where they are and also have a vague feeling this is not where they want to stay. If you are in this group, take heart. You can still get out and go for the gold in your life.

The people who make it happen may hit bouts of short-term burnout, but they don't stay there. They don't wallow in doubt or apathy. This is a relatively small group in modern society. They aren't content with mediocrity. This group starts businesses, creates organizations to better their community, builds buildings, and takes risks. If they fail, and they often do, they pick themselves back up again and keep going until they succeed. They don't feel sorry for themselves and don't wait on someone else to rescue them. They take initiative when most others are taking the safe route.

Tip: Don't fall for the falsehood that only Alpha personalities with a special gift for success can belong to this group. If you are serious about breaking out of burnout and are still breathing, you have hope.

If you're stuck in burnout, take a breath, and take your pulse. If you have a pulse, that means that you can get out of burnout, and come back stronger than ever. You can become a person who makes it happen. Think about how you arrived at this point. Are you stuck in a job you hate? Have you spent the last 15 years pouring energy into your children only to realize you haven't poured any into yourself? Do you have a dream that you haven't chased because you're too busy living someone else's dream?

If so, I've got good news and bad news. First, the good news. You can most definitely break out of burnout. You can build a meaningful life, and become a person who makes it happen in your world. You can once again wake up excited to face the day and make a difference.

Now, the bad news. **This is where we break with conventional wisdom on burnout.** Conventional wisdom places the responsibility of solving employee burnout on the employer. We place the responsibility on the individual. *If you are waiting for your supervisor to become an angel and rescue you from the malaise of burnout, you may be in for a long wait.*

You may say, "but you don't understand what I'm up against at work." Point taken. I have not walked in your shoes. But I have walked in mine. I've burned out on jobs and burned out in life. Burnout is both a warning and an opportunity. It's a warning that something is wrong, but also an opportunity to make things right. Your boss will never be perfect. You can't change your supervisor, or your spouse, or your kids. The only person you can change is yourself.

On the home front, don't look to your spouse or family. Family dynamics have a powerful influence on our happiness, but just like with your boss, don't wait for family to take the initiative to change you. Do it yourself, and let them see the change over time. One big difference between family and work: You can change jobs, but changing family is a different matter. I can't quit my kids or walk away from my elderly mother. When my brother had cancer, we couldn't give up on him. When facing family pressures that may for a season take you under water, realize it won't last forever. When you come back up for air, carve out ways to work on yourself.

If you've been a person who watched life happen, you can become a person who makes life happen. It takes a paradigm shift followed by action. Don't worry about the folks who wonder what happened. They aren't reading this book. Concern yourself with becoming a person who makes it happen.

A person who makes it happen takes control of life and accepts responsibility for moving forward. This involves owning up to your situation and putting together a plan for moving forward. But before we drill into the specifics of a personal plan for breaking out of burnout, let's take a moment to consider a big part of the puzzle.

CHAPTER 5

IT'S YOUR PROBLEM—OWN IT

Our human response to a problem like burnout is to blame someone, something, anything other than ourselves. ***Stop it!*** (As a symbolic exercise, put your book down for a moment, take one hand, and give yourself a slight slap on the other wrist.)

The big three of family, friends, and co-workers are too busy with their own problems to drive your "breaking out of burnout" train. While we can and will investigate some key societal and workplace pressures surrounding burnout, realize that you cannot fix burnout by changing the world around you. However, you can begin changing your own world. The first step in this process is accepting ownership of your burnout.

You alone are responsible for correcting your current situation. Blaming others will not change your situation one iota. There's something liberating in saying to yourself, "It's my problem and I'm going to do something about it, starting right now!" Now that we've established that the responsibility for breaking out of burnout lies with you, it's okay to step back and take a peek at the burnout big picture.

Institutional burnout runs rampant in today's world. Any profession or situation in life that requires constant contact with people needing your attention is prime for burnout. However, it is not the scope of this book to attempt to cure institutional burnout. Our goal is to provide insight and practical tools to help you overcome burnout and come back stronger. This starts with a major personal attitude makeover.

Burnout produces passivity, causing you to feel oppressed by an invisible force beyond your control. You want to change, but too often feel powerless to change it. This points to the very paradigm shift that must take place in order to move forward. You must realize that ***you change the world by first changing yourself.***

You may say, "But my supervisor is just too unreasonable." If you work in an institutional setting, chances are your supervisor may be burned out, too. Just as one drowning person can't save another, neither can one burned-out person rescue another. Don't let a difficult supervisor or co-worker keep you stuck in burnout.

Let's cough up another hairball. The burnout is your fault. You allowed it to happen by allowing others to rule your agenda. Even as I write these words, other people demand a piece of my time. *Do you have some time to meet this week? It won't take long. Can you please return my phone call? I only need a minute. Will you attend my conference? It will be so uplifting for you. I sent you an email this morning and haven't heard back yet. What's up?*

Some of these things we simply must do. But the decision to relegate our lives to the demands of others is ours alone to make. People pleasers too often end up pleasing everyone but themselves. Overcoming burnout requires a paradigm shift of viewing life through the lenses of your priorities. This sounds selfish, but it's actually the opposite. You have much more to offer those who seek your time if you possess wisdom and understanding from pursuing your own development. ***If you burn out, you cannot be a***

light to those around you.
How do you deal with all life's interruptions without becoming bitter and resentful toward those seeking your time? You combat the sources of burnout by building a life based on your priorities and goals. The best way to beat burnout is by developing a great life.

Here's one thing you should remember. Nobody else is going to overcome burnout for you. Not your supervisor, not your Human Resources Director, not your spouse, nor your best friend. Your kids won't do it. The person wanting the phone call returned won't do it. I'm not saying they don't need you. I'm saying they won't dig you out of the hole. *The only person who can break you out of burnout is the one staring at you in the mirror.*

Here's another pill to swallow. Stop feeling sorry for yourself. Burnout produces self-pity along with passivity. A person in burn-out mode turns inward and begins to see the world through the dark glasses of what "they are doing to me." This only makes the situation worse. A person at this stage may turn to alcohol, overeating, or other unhealthy habits to medicate emotional pain. Self-pity also leads to isolation. Most people in burn-out mode think they are the only one with a problem.

I saw an old buddy recently and asked how things were going. "Everything is busy but good," he replied. We proceeded to chat about how life gets busier as we get older. I agreed with his sentiment that life is good but busy. Yet, allow me to translate.

"My life is really busy. I thought by this stage things would slow down, but they haven't. I've got problems. Real problems. I'm too scared to tell you about them because I'm sure you've got it all together, and I don't want you to think I'm struggling." We run into someone at the store, the ball game, or at church, and the banter begins. "How are things going?" "Great." Then we silently ponder "if they only knew."

The Greek word *hupocritos* means "one who wears a mask." In ancient Greek plays, actors would put on a mask to show emotion. A smiling mask meant they were happy. A mask with a frown meant they were sad. From this, we get the English word "hypocrite" to denote someone who pretends to be something in public that they are not in private. Those in burnout often develop a hypocritical view of life. They may complain to a couple of close friends, but they pretend everything is "just great" to everyone else.

If not reversed, the influences involved in wearing a mask turn into anger and bitterness. At this point, someone in burnout is just plain miserable. They're putting on an act to make it through the day and trying to get to the weekend of mindless movies, alcohol, or sleeping till noon.

While such methods may provide a temporary break from the monotony of burnout, prolonged use as a crutch will only make matters worse. A temporary escape from burnout through the use of unhealthy habits compounds the problem. What's worse than being burned out? Being burned out, drunk, and hungover. Not everyone battling burnout becomes a junkie, but many develop unhealthy coping habits.

A word about victim mentality. When battling burnout, victim mentality is toxic. Progress can't take place if you see yourself as a "victim" of the boss, the system, the man, or whoever. When breaking out of burnout, you'll be too busy doing positive things to dwell on the negative. A victim is generally viewed as powerless over the cause of his or her injury or harm. You will never move forward if you see yourself as powerless over the burnout in your life.

That's why an attitude adjustment must take place. Look at it this way. You are the CEO of a one-person company. That person is you. Your destiny is in your hands. This doesn't mean that you are some hot shot who can tell everyone else to take a hike. It means that you are ultimately the only human truly in charge of your life. Outside of God, no one on this earth is more interested in your own well-being than *you*. No one else will look out for your best interest like you.

I am the CEO of a non-profit organization. I spend most of my energy on the job interacting with people either through face-to-face meetings, phone, email, or letters. Sometimes I make decisions that are not in the short-term interest of a particular individual. That's because, at the end of the day, my job is to look out for the best interest of the organization rather than the interest of any one person.

It's the same way with you. As the CEO of a one-person company, you are tasked with looking out for your own best interests. When burned out, you are definitely not looking out for your personal best interests. Burnout happens when you consistently put your own interests on the back burner to bail out other people.

It sounds selfish to say "I'm the CEO of a one-person company. ME." Heck, it sounds selfish to write it. But here's the underlying truth. If you burn out, you ultimately hurt not only yourself but also the people who you are tasked with helping. A burned-out mom short-changes her kids. A burned-out counselor short-changes his clients. A burned-out doctor short-changes her patients. A burned-out adult child short-changes an elderly parent, and the list goes on.

Tip: Don't proclaim to the world, "I've read a book and now I'm the CEO of my own one-person company! Get out of my face!"

People don't want to hear that. Just start privately living each day as your own CEO. Focus on your own priorities for a change rather than someone else's.

The most selfless thing you can do for those who depend on you is to be the best person you can be. In the interest of self-disclosure, I'm fiercely individualistic. I believe strongly in the rights of an individual to lead the life he or she chooses, as long as it is legal, moral, and ethical. Now, a few pointers on this new attitude.

Pointer one: This will feel weird at first. Burnout produces a feeling of emotional insecurity. It gives rise to the concept deep inside that we are faulty and not worthy of esteem. Our ideas won't work. Nobody will listen to us. For sure, we all have our quirks and hang-ups. But the rich and powerful have hang-ups too. They just don't let their quirks stop them from barreling ahead and living life to the fullest.

When you step out and begin to live confidently, it will feel strange at first. Sort of like the athlete on the 30-30-30 team who rides the bench. (Only gets put in when the team is 30 points ahead or 30 points behind with 30 seconds to go.) When you're suddenly thrown into the game, you don't quite know what to do, so you jack up an airball from 30 feet out or dribble the ball off your foot and out of bounds.

A person beaten down by burnout will feel strange when suddenly taking even a small step toward self-fulfillment. Yet, taken properly that step can be exhilarating. Start saying to yourself, "I can do this! I can do this!" Changing your personal mindset is the most important part of breaking out of burnout.

How do you change your mindset? How do you go from accepting responsibility to actually doing something about it when your brain screams, "You can't do it!!" Here's another little secret. You've got to change the way you act in order to get a different outcome. You can read books, go to counselors, have hands laid on you at church, watch motivational videos, curse burnout to its face, and feel groovy about your new direction. But nothing will change until you take an action. Let me preach on it. *You change behavior by changing your behavior.*

You've simply got to act your way to a new way of thinking. If you're like Elvis and crave jelly doughnuts, and wake up one day 30 pounds heavier, you're going to have to put down the doughnuts and start exercising to get healthy. It just doesn't work to wait longingly for the day you no longer crave the sweet taste of a jelly doughnut crossing your eagerly awaiting lips. That day will never come.

Let me repeat. ***You've got to act your way to a new way of thinking.*** Start with one thing. Maybe an exercise program or reading 30 minutes a day. Start with one positive new thing that you control, and do it daily until it becomes a habit. Developing positive new habits is vital to overcoming burnout.

Now that we've established that you must take ownership of your breaking out of burnout journey, we're almost ready to get underway. Almost. First, understand that you've got to be ready to start this journey. If you want to win the heart of a new romantic interest, you don't go on a first date without showering and cleaning up to look your best.

Answering the doorbell looking like a slob and starting the conversation about how you are unemployed and have no plans to work will likely steal any hope of a budding, new relationship. In the same way, we will now look at some major issues that drain the energy to break out of burnout.

CHAPTER SIX
HOPE STEALERS

Long ago and far away, I invited a young lady to my apartment for dinner. After she arrived, we sat down on my bachelor pad couch for light conversation. No sooner had we started talking when I looked in horror near the front door and saw where my cat had taken a nice, fresh dump on the brown carpet. There it lay in plain sight, right in front of me and my date. Unfortunately, I had not performed a last-minute inspection, and this relationship was doomed from the beginning due to my oversight.

We can jaw on the front porch of life about breaking out of burnout until Mr. Clean grows hair, but certain factors can torpedo your journey if unaddressed. I call these factors hope stealers because they rob hope and joy from your life. If you don't wrestle in these areas, consider yourself blessed. Sit back, read this chapter, and learn something. But if you do, please take a time-out to work on these areas.

A person burned out in life needs hope. But as we age, multiple problems can arise at the same time. If you're only burned out on the job, the journey is straightforward. However, people in burnout often find themselves dealing with multiple problems. Burnout combined with a bad marriage, an addiction, health problems, or a bad attitude presents a double whammy.

Let's start with marriage. If you are burned out on your job and *also* trapped in a failing marriage, your marital problems will throw cold water on any attempts to improve the job situation. Studies show a bad marriage to be a major contributor to people who fail in life. By failure, I mean people who don't achieve their goals or life dreams.

A note about marriage. Don't use Hollywood or politics as your textbook on marriage. We all know a rock star on his fifth marriage or a tomcat business tycoon who ranks among the rich and powerful. No matter how successful a person may appear, a bad marriage will drain energy from his or her success.

One of the most important decisions you will make in life is choosing a marital spouse. Choose the right person, and your joys will be multiplied. Choose the wrong person, and your sorrows will be multiplied. If you are trapped in a bad marriage, talk to your spouse, and try to get help. Know that your marriage will be like the proverbial ball and chain until you deal with it.

Studies show a direct correlation between healthy marriages and burnout levels. People involved in healthy marriages are less likely to succumb permanently to chronic burnout. Conversely, people in unhealthy marriages are more likely to experience chronic burnout. This doesn't mean you have to be Ward and June Cleaver to avoid burnout. Rather, it points to the drag a failing marriage will put on attempts to overcome career burnout.

If your co-workers are your only social outlet, your social life can become an extension of water cooler complaints about the boss. Getting the kids to soccer practice gets you involved in something other than your own problems. I didn't notice burnout in my own life while the kids were in high school, as being involved in their activities provided a life outside the workplace that did not revolve around me.

A good marriage also provides someone with whom to talk through work problems and experience positive activities outside of work. It is entirely possible to have a good marriage and great family and still experience burnout. You can be content in your life and be single. However, studies show that people in problematic marriages run a greater risk of not pulling out of burnout if it strikes.

Another note about marriage. You can have a wonderful marriage and still crash and burn in your job or career. However, a decent marriage provides a partner who will stick by your side as you work through your issues and encourage you along the journey.

Crippling Addictions

We all have bad or annoying habits. It's part of being human. However, the wrong habits can capsize your boat and make digging out of burnout more difficult. As John Maxwell says, "Too many people are trying to go uphill with downhill habits."

Yet, another category of unhealthy behavior goes beyond mere bad habits like watching too much television or drinking too much diet soda. These *crippling addictions* carry the potential to destroy your quality of life.

Let's start with alcohol. A 2006 study by the Finnish Institute of Occupational Health found a direct link between burnout and alcohol dependence. Though the study did not link burnout with high consumption rates, it did point to an increase in alcohol dependency among employees complaining of burnout. Job stress carries an increased risk for habitual alcohol use as a relief mechanism for burnout.

Growing numbers of people also use prescription medications to numb burnout. Studies show 19 million Americans abused prescription medications in 2016 alone. While medications such as pain pills, tranquilizers, anti-anxiety drugs, and stimulants have specific benefits when properly prescribed and used, they can slow down or extinguish efforts to overcome burnout if abused.

If you struggle with burnout, realize that engaging in addictive behavior will only make things worse. If you are burned out and also deal with a full-blown addiction such as chronic alcoholism, please get help in dealing with your addiction. Efforts to overcome burnout will not succeed if you don't also conquer the addictive behavior.

Health Issues

My father was the best daddy a kid could have. He taught me to mow the grass, dig a post hole, work a garden, and catch catfish. He was a loving grandfather to my daughters. He died at 76 from congestive heart failure. A few months before he died, he took the oxygen cable out of his nose, turned to my daughters and said, "Girls, whatever you do, don't smoke cigarettes." Smoking was my dad's one and only vice. It took him to the grave.

Everyone develops certain health problems during the aging process. It's part of life. Arthritis, acid reflux, high blood pressure, migraines, diabetes, joint and back pain are just a few examples. We can learn to manage these symptoms through proper medication, diet, and exercise. While such maladies may cause temporary setbacks, they need not hinder a full life if properly handled.

However, there comes a point where losing one's health can end the ability to live out personal hopes and dreams. Visit a hospital, nursing home, or hospice facility, and you will see people who are still alive but have lost all ability to live their dream. That's why it's imperative to take care of yourself while you still have your health.

The large majority of America's health budget is spent on five areas, which are all within our control. Too much stress, too much smoking, too much alcohol, improper diet, and not enough exercise. None of us can cheat Father Time, but we don't have to help him rush the process.

Any effort to overcome burnout will be significantly hampered by an unhealthy lifestyle. We've all heard the stories of "Grandpa," who rolled his own cigarettes, drank a gallon of white lightning every day, ate fatback all his life, and lived to be 103 years old. Such stories make for a good laugh, but they don't make good sense. (These folks often have a second story about their third cousin who ate seaweed, ran marathons, never touched a cigarette or a bottle, and dropped dead of a heart attack at 42 years old.)

When it comes to your health, don't take chances. Odds are if you eat a balanced diet, get moderate exercise, don't smoke cigarettes, and moderate your alcohol intake, you'll live a longer, healthier life than if you spend your life smoking, drinking, and gorging at the all-you-can-eat buffet.

If you find yourself in burnout mode, check your lifestyle. Nobody starts on an unhealthy path thinking it will kill them. Our human nature tells us that we'll change before it's too late. However, too many people never make that change. Don't wait until you get a fatal diagnosis.

Apathy

Apathy is perhaps the greatest hope stealer of them all. A person who is apathetic has burned out and quit caring. This individual has lost all zest for life and would rather spend time complaining and making everyone else's life miserable than doing something about it.

Ignorance can be overcome through learning. Marriages can be restored if both spouses are willing to work through differences. Addictions can be conquered if the individual is willing to stop the addictive behavior and work toward recovery. Vigor can often be regained through healthy living, modern medicine, and proper medication. But if you have given up, it's a lost cause as long as you wallow in apathy.

According to Newton's First Law of Motion, *an object at rest stays at rest, and an object in motion stays in motion with the same speed and in the same direction unless acted upon by an unbalanced force.*

If you are burned out, don't give up. However, don't curse fate because you haven't won the lottery. If you're sitting on your butt and burned out, you'll continue sitting on your butt until you act on your situation with an unbalanced force. For example, you get up and start a new routine. At some point, everyone stuck in burnout realizes John Wayne is not going to ride to their rescue, yank them off their couch, refill their gas tank, stick a lollipop in their mouth, and blaze a new trail for them.

Apathy is always at hand. It whispers in our ear, "You don't matter. You can't do it. Why bother?" One key difference between successful and unsuccessful people is that successful people outrun apathy. They hear the same voice, but tune it out and replace it with affirming messages such as, "I can and will do this. I can and will make a difference. I'm here for a reason."

The saddest thing I've witnessed in life is grown, healthy people who have given up. They slump through life, wanting others to fix their problems and blaming others when they don't. *If you attempt nothing, you will accomplish nothing.*

I took a computer programming class in college back before the days of Windows. You had to enter cryptic commands onto a blank screen, input your data, and then print your work on a dot-matrix printer. My first attempts failed. I entered my data, hit the command button, but nothing happened. Nada. Not a thing.

With the help of an instructor, I retraced my steps and realized the error of not entering a character necessary to execute the program. I fixed the error and successfully completed the project. This was my initiation into the concept of GIGO, or "garbage in, garbage out."

Tip: You don't have to victoriously conquer all areas of personal shortcoming before beginning your fight against burnout. However, you do need to be aware of the major issues that will sabotage your efforts if unaddressed.

We don't go to bed passionate and wake up apathetic. We become apathetic after a long period of putting garbage into our minds and bodies. To reverse this process, you must change what you put into your mind. Let's now move to that step.

In moving to this next step, understand that once awakened to the fact that you are burned out, you can no longer claim ignorance. Gone are the uneasy days of feeling that something isn't right but not knowing what to call it. This means you are now compelled to do something about the burnout monster lurking under your bed.

PART 2
THE GREAT AWAKENING

The alarm goes off at 5:00 a.m. You hit snooze and roll over for eight more minutes of sleep. About the time you doze back off, the alarm goes off again. You're torn, not ready to crawl out from under the warm blankets, but you also know that you can't just lay there and sleep the morning away if you want to get anything done. You must take that inevitable step of throwing off the covers and getting out of bed to hit the shower. Once out of the shower and dressed, you're wide awake and charging out the door.

Likewise, when awakening from burnout, there comes a moment of decision. You can no longer ignore the reality of your situation, but it's hard to get your emotional muscles and bones going in a new direction. Familiarity, even if grounded in misery, can provide a perverse comfort.

Yet, you're now fully awake to the fact that the old life and routine no longer work. It's time to get out of bed and face a new day. You may not know what to do next, but you know you can't sleep your life away in bed. You're awake in a new life, and it's time to hit the shower.

CHAPTER SEVEN

NO EXCUSES

On Sunday morning, February 13th, 2011, I lined up for the starting gun of the New Orleans Rock and Roll Marathon/Half Marathon. Frank Shorter, the winner of the 1972 Olympic marathon in Munich, Germany was the master of ceremonies. The morning dawned sunny and 47 degrees, perfect running weather. Shorter took the microphone and challenged the runners, saying "This is a no excuses day." Great running weather plus a flat course means, in runner lingo, that you can't blame the weather or the course for not having your best day.

I had trained for the half-marathon with intervals of jogging four minutes and walking one minute. However, I also wanted to run a personal best. About three miles into the race, I realized that if this race was to produce a personal record, I would have to forgo the one-minute walk breaks and run the entire remaining 10 miles without walk breaks.

Shorter's challenge rang through my mind: "This is a no excuses day!" I kicked it in, ran the remaining 10 miles of the race, and set a personal best in the half marathon of two hours and 15 minutes. That's slow by racing standards, but lightning fast for me. I'll never forget that day and will be forever thankful for the "no excuses" challenge. Without it, I would have settled for less than my best.

Our human nature tends to blame something besides ourselves for personal problems. However, when dealing with burnout, excuses don't help. You can scream till doomsday about how you could get it together if not for the workplace, the boss, the government, the system, or family responsibilities. However, all you'll get is a sore throat.

The moon and stars will never line up perfectly for you. There will never be a "right" time to start a new approach. So, why not start today? Waiting until the "right time" is a dream killer. Saying, "I hate my job but I can't do anything about it right now because the kids are in school" will only postpone the inevitable crash.

Entitlement mentality is a first cousin to excuses. Many have come to believe that good fortune should just happen. Contrary to what we hear in popular culture, life doesn't award participation trophies. An award for playing the game may make little Johnny feel appreciated, but it doesn't teach him that hard work precedes accomplishment.

Everyone in New Orleans awoke to sunny skies and 47 degrees on February 13th, 2011. However, not everybody was in shape to run a race. The runners still had to put in the months of jogging, stretching, and long training runs to be prepared for the "no excuses" day. You may be able to walk a 5K with little preparation, but, if you want to win in life's marathon, you must do the solitary hard work of preparation.

It's hard to get up early on a Saturday morning to run eight miles alone. It's hard to get up before work to jog or to come home after work, and put in a three miler. However, if you don't do the work, you won't be ready when the "no excuses" moment arrives.

Participation-trophy mentality instills the wrong ethic. It teaches that we are owed success simply because we breathe. News Flash! You will never reach your personal best with participation-trophy mentality. If you're stuck in burnout mode, stop making excuses, and realize that you're going to have to do the work to get back in shape.

Facing significant challenges is part of the human experience. Whether you are among the rich and famous or poor and anonymous, you will face trials in this life. At times, you will have to go into crisis mode to deal with problems, such as the sickness of a family member or ripping up the soaked carpet from a water line leak.

However, most of the demons that send us into burnout mode are not crisis oriented. We feel stuck because our boss is a jerk or because the paycheck doesn't cover the bills. Our dream job turns into a nightmare. When burned out, it's your responsibility to start the process of rebuilding your life. No one else will do it for you.

I've learned the hard way that, unless I want to part with the cash and pay someone else to do the job, my grass won't mow itself. My clothes won't wash themselves. The food in the freezer won't jump onto the stove and cook itself. In the same way, no one will do the hard work for you of restarting your engine.

Be careful where you look for answers. Someone who has never burned out may offer advice, but will not understand your situation. Burnout may be rampant in some professions, but don't assume that everybody burns out.

People with high ideals and lofty goals are prime candidates for burnout. Those who start their career with a strong desire to "change the world" or "make the world a better place" often enter a profession that calls for helping people in need. When the reality of a not so perfect workplace combines with the fact that not everybody can be rescued, it often produces disillusionment that leads to burnout. At this point, conscientious employees who started out with noble intentions of helping people can adopt a cynical, cold view of the very people they start out trying to help.

The teacher who began a career hoping to educate young minds can become embittered toward students, seeing them as spoiled brats. The pastor who started off wanting to nourish souls can come to view parishioners as spiritually shallow. The counselor who felt a calling to help addicts can begin to see them as unwilling to change. The pharmacist who wanted to help people take their proper medications can devolve into someone who sees patients as too stupid to follow instructions.

Tip: Not everybody burns out.

Low achievers are not a high-risk category for burnout, nor are people who don't have high aspirations. Freudenberger limits burnout to "dynamic, charismatic, goal-oriented men and women or to determined idealists." These people want to have the best careers, marriages, and have high self and community expectations and ideals.

Yet, life is not perfect and people with high aspirations are prime candidates for burnout when those dreams go unfulfilled. These people are not happy with average jobs because their internal messaging says they should aim for the stars and settle for nothing less. So, if you aim for the stars and only hit the moon, you may see yourself as a failure. Whether working as a nurse or an executive, anything short of top-flight success doesn't cut it.

Rather than expecting to toil away at the factory like their parent's generation, this group grew up thinking they would change the world and leave a mark. When the grind of life exerts its inevitable pressure, these idealists can go into a form of shock that culminates in burnout.

If you feel burned out, take courage. That means you want to change your world. It means you want to leave your world better than you found it. If so, quit making excuses, and get ready to finish strong in the life you've been given.

This is where the fun begins. With negative self-talk in the rear-view mirror, it's time to examine your strengths and passions. This is where the discipline begins of making sure you spend time each day doing some things you enjoy. It's where the journey of "doing the daily work" begins to get you in shape for breaking out of burnout.

CHAPTER EIGHT

WHERE TO START

If burnout is a drag, doing positive things we enjoy is the opposite. These things excite us and provide a compelling reason to get out of bed each morning. Identifying your passions and strengths gives you the "it" factor in overcoming burnout.

You don't just wake up from a long span of burnout, throw open the curtains to allow the morning light to pour in, and declare "good morning world. I now love my life and am no longer burned out!" If only it were that easy.

Allow me a moment of author's privilege. I believe we are created by God and endowed with a unique purpose for our life on this earth. Burnout is not our proverbial "cross to bear." Rather, it is a wake-up call to prepare us for the next chapter in life. If not for burnout, no one would go back to school in their forties. We'd keep our first job out of college. Stale marriages wouldn't improve. Second careers wouldn't be launched. People in their fifties wouldn't train for their first triathlon. Second-half of life bucket lists would never have items checked off.

Burnout is the nerve pain of our emotional system. It alerts us that something is wrong. At first, we ignore the pain or think it will go away. However, it only gets worse until we finally take healing action and bring ourselves back into a state of wellness.

When physically ill, a trip to the doctor's office leads to an examination of the symptoms. Our blood pressure, temperature, and weight are all checked. The doctor may listen to our heartbeat, breathing, and look into eyes and ears to determine a diagnosis and course of corrective action.

Likewise, a personal examination is a good start to overcoming burnout. Evaluate your strengths. Get a pen and paper and ask yourself the following questions.

- What am I good at?
- What do I enjoy doing?
- What are my strengths?
- What are my personal areas of giftedness and talent?
- What are my dreams?
- What resources can I bring to bear in pursuit of hopes, dreams, and life goals?

Tip: Handwriting uses a part of the brain that typing does not. Writing out your self-evaluation brings out your best ideas and cements them into your mind.

A written self-evaluation of your personal strengths puts you in the driver's seat. Whereas burnout puts the focus on your weaknesses, an examination of your personal strengths and talents places the focus on your potential. Developing your strengths is critical to overcoming burnout. It's also much more enjoyable working on what you enjoy and do well, as opposed to consuming your energy on unpleasant or boring tasks.

Burned out people spend a lot of time doing things they don't like. Over an extended period of time, job requirements and life responsibilities force people into certain molds. Parents may love their children, but the daily requirements of getting kids to school, soccer practice, t-ball, band, or similar activities turn into a daily grind. A doctor loves the job, but didn't bargain for the endless paperwork involved in keeping patient records.

A teacher who dreamed of educating young minds never foresaw the draining monotony of maintaining order among thirty noisy students. A public defender with a heart for justice among members of the underclass becomes disillusioned at having to defend guilty offenders. The mid-level salesperson who worked hard for an executive level promotion didn't reckon for the new loads of paperwork and meetings.

In order to reverse the pattern of doing what you don't like, it's important to also examine your passions. What excites you and gets your adrenaline pumping? What stirs your soul and makes you want to get up in the morning? Your strengths and passions give strong hints as to where to exert your main focus. Whether a job or a hobby, when you start working toward a goal that utilizes your natural talents and captures your passion, you are well on your way toward breaking out of burnout.

Passions can change as we age. The passion to find a spouse or buy your first home may be strong in your twenties, but a distant memory at 45. External voices and pressures often say stick with your activities, passions, and careers of yesterday. However, burnout will not be cured by yesterday's routine. Remember, you're burned out doing what you did yesterday, and you'll stay burned out if you keep doing it.

In college, I could eat the legs off the table and weigh a steady 160 pounds. Large pizzas, all-you-can-eat buffets, and grandma's home cooking couldn't put another pound on my skinny frame. Therefore, a balanced diet was not a passion at that stage of life. Fast forward to my mid-30s, and I noticed the pants were fitting tighter around the waist than before. One day I stepped on the scales, and the dial came to rest on 194 pounds. At that point, watching what I eat became a passion. While I've never returned to my beanpole days, balanced eating became a focus, as I grew older.

Tip: You will not burnout working toward something that excites you.

Therefore, it's important in the early battle against burnout to get a small victory under your belt. Nothing ignites momentum like winning. Pick a doable, two-sided goal. On one side, it should be doable. On the other side, it should stretch you a bit. What type of goal should you set? While that answer lies within you, let's examine a time held truth.

A man on a discussion panel was once asked what changed his life. "I took up running," he responded. The moderator astutely observed that when we take a step in the physical, a positive result often happens in the spiritual. Obedience precedes the miracle. In the Old Testament, the Israelite priests had to first put their foot in the waters of the flood-swollen Jordan River before the waters parted. The Syrian General Naaman had to dip in the Jordan River seven times before his leprosy disappeared. In the same way, when overcoming burnout, a step in the physical realm often leads to a breakthrough in the spiritual or emotional realm.

Jog or walk a 5k, lose 10 pounds, or sign up and complete a fitness class. These types of short-term wins provide momentum for a new life. A short-term win can also be cleaning out the garage, reading that book you bought last year, or attending a personal improvement seminar. The key lies in completing a positive step that excites you and gets you going in the right direction. The accomplishment of completing 25 consecutive push-ups when you couldn't do any one month before proves that you can accomplish more than you thought. Completing 25 push-ups may be a stretch starting from scratch, but it's doable within a few weeks.

Also, examine your personality. You can't change your personality, but it's important to understand your basic personality type. Many different tests exist, ranging from quick online surveys to expensive tests that drill deep into your psyche. For our purposes, an internet search can reveal numerous free tests that only take a few minutes.

Are you extroverted or introverted? This doesn't necessarily mean you are outgoing or shy. Introverts can be social and extroverts can be dis-engaging at times. In terms of understanding your personality, extroverts recharge their emotional batteries by talking to others. Introverts recharge their emotional batteries by withdrawing to themselves. When extroverts need to recharge, they must find someone to talk to. As they talk, they charge their batteries. When introverts need to recharge, they must get alone and withdraw to their cave.

I recently chatted with an introverted friend who has an extroverted roommate. The roommate scheduled an out-of-town trip, and my friend looked forward to a quiet weekend alone to recharge her batteries. She came home to surprisingly find her roommate sitting on the couch, excitedly telling her, "I just didn't feel right about leaving you alone all weekend. Let's watch a movie together!"

Understanding whether you are the person who needs to crawl into a cave after a busy day or talk through your day with another human being is key. Both extroverts and introverts can burn out, but they'll likely process it differently.

For personality discussions, I find the animal analogies easy to understand. You don't have to be a psychologist to relate to the Lion, Golden Retriever, Otter, and Beaver. A lion is the take charge person always in command. The lion is king of the jungle and wants everyone to know it. Lions make quick decisions and will tell you what they think. Lions instinctively take initiative and don't often ask for permission.

The golden retriever is the loyal, good-natured friend. They are easy to get along with and don't like conflict. Golden retrievers make good team members and will often wait for others to speak before stating their opinion.

The otter is the socializer of the group. Otters never miss a chance to turn an occasion into a party. They love to have fun and make friends quickly. Otters have a good time and want to involve others in the festivities they create.

Beavers are the process-oriented thinkers and planners of the group. Beavers don't do anything without first planning it out. They are methodical with a bent toward detail. Beavers often play the "devil's advocate" role and point out problems that must be solved before moving forward.

Most people are a mix of these types, with one dominant personality type and a strong secondary type. For example, a person can primarily be a take-charge lion, with a strong secondary otter personality. This person will plan the lunch party, decide who gets invited, assign the seating, and make sure everyone has a good time.

However, all personality types have weaknesses. A lion can be blind to the feelings of a conflict-averse golden retriever. A beaver may throw a wrench into a worthy project if its process isn't followed. A golden retriever can turn stubborn if she feels ignored. The otter can use charm to get information and then become the office gossip.

In dealing with burnout, understanding your personality helps explain how you react to certain situations and how others react to you. A burned-out golden retriever may seethe internally when aversion to conflict is too often mistaken for agreement and explode unexpectedly. A fun-loving otter may go into depression when constantly overwhelmed by the needs of clients, patients, or customers in the workplace.

A burned-out lion can shut down and quit making decisions after too many conflicts with burned-out golden retrievers who have morphed into stubborn mules. A burned-out beaver can create a workplace logjam by insisting that the process is more important than the outcome.

People in burnout are often not assertive and let others control their lives and time. The dictates of the job, the stress of raising a family, or the needs of elderly parents can create a life of putting the needs of others before your own needs. This creates a classic burnout scenario. Bitterness turns to anger, which then turns to apathy.

Not every factor leading to burnout can be addressed at once. It's not wise to walk away from a job that pays the bills if you don't have another career lined up. (There can be an exception if you face long-term workplace abuse or are asked to engage in unethical or illegal behavior. If you're asked to do something illegal or unethical by your employer, don't do it. Your employer might try to hang the rap on you if things go south.)

So, start with a small win. GET A HOBBY! People go fishing and kayaking for a reason. They enjoy something that provides a break from the workplace routine. It may not be feasible to change jobs or careers right now. A burned-out mom can't tell her kids to take a hike instead of taking them to school. However, you can carve out a hobby for yourself. Join a book club, play bunco, take guitar lessons, or join a hunting club.

Tip: When it comes to hobbies, the internet is your friend.

Name a subject, and you can find an online class or a YouTube tutorial about it. Most of these tutorials are free, and you can watch them at your convenience. If you've always wanted to become a backyard car mechanic or sushi chef, there's a cornucopia of online videos on subjects that will interest you.

Too many burned out people say, "But I don't have time for myself." They toil, day in and day out, with the mindset of the old spiritual song that says "nobody knows the trouble I've seen." Developing a hobby reverses that mindset through an activity that engages the body and mind intentionally doing something you enjoy.

Picture your bank account. For financial health, you have to deposit more money into your bank account than you withdraw. You certainly have to make withdrawals in the form of utility bills, the mortgage, and buying groceries. However, if you don't deposit more money into your account than you withdraw, you'll wind up in debt.

By the time someone burns out, they've spent several years withdrawing more from their emotional bank account than they deposited. By this time, the single deposit of a quick summer vacation or night out with the girls won't put your emotional bank account back in order. People too often try to cure burnout with the single deposit of a week off at the beach. While that can help temporarily, it won't solve the problem if you return to the unhealthy practice of withdrawing more emotionally than you deposit after the vacation is over.

Take that same person with an overdrawn bank account and maxed out credit cards. Give them the small win of saving $1,000.00 in cash for an emergency fund, and they can see light at the end of the tunnel.

Likewise, if you can create a small win of depositing 30 minutes a day doing something you enjoy into your emotional bank account, you can see the light at the end of the burnout tunnel. You're not there yet, but the fact that you took a 30-minute walk provides hope.

Start with 30 minutes a day that you set aside for "me time." Whether this is exercising at first light, journaling, or reading 30 minutes before bed, do it consistently. Make the daily deposit into your emotional bank account. If you miss a day, don't quit or beat yourself up. Just jump back in the game the next day.

When you start a new hobby or a positive daily routine, you'll most certainly miss a day. It happens to everyone. How you react is critical. Successful people learn how to jump back in the next day and get back on track. Unsuccessful people don't. Which group you join is up to you.

Don't ignore your spiritual condition when taking this journey. Burnout can be God's way of getting your attention because He's about to do a new work in your life. Therefore, seek God in the depths of burnout for spiritual wholeness.

With burnout, God is there, even when we don't feel a Divine presence. However, don't rely on pithy sermons or well-meaning people who tell you to pray more or read your Bible cover to cover. Nothing is wrong with those things, but religious ritual will not heal the scars of burnout. Learn to listen for God in the quiet moments of your hectic, busy life. Set aside a few minutes each day to meditate, journal, and ask God simply to speak to your soul.

Evaluate yourself, develop a hobby, and listen for the Divine voice in your soul. Now that you've examined areas of strength and passion and started some positive activities to bring energy to your day, realize that you've got to change the messaging in your head.

Listening to the wrong messages, or worse yet, no messages at all, will make sure your journey out of burnout hits a sure-fire dead end. Listening to the right messages can save your life.

CHAPTER 9
LISTENING TO THE RIGHT MESSAGE

In August 2005, National Weather Service Meteorologist Robert Ricks kept watch over a strengthening Hurricane Katrina. As the storm approached the Louisiana/Mississippi coast, Ricks wrote a weather bulletin issued on August 28th outlining the storm's catastrophic punch. Realizing the bulletin contained frightening language, Ricks began looking for sentences to delete but concluded the contents were accurate and left them intact. Known today simply as "The Bulletin," Rick's bulletin and the rosary he clutched while riding out Hurricane Katrina are enshrined in the National Museum of American History.

000
WWUS74 KLIX 281550
NPWLIX

URGENT — WEATHER MESSAGE
NATIONAL WEATHER SERVICENEW ORLEANSLA
1011 AM CDTSUN AUG 28, 2005

...DEVASTATING DAMAGE EXPECTED...
HURRICANE KATRINA...A MOST POWERFUL HURRICANE WITH UNPRECEDENTED STRENGTH... RIVALING THE INTENSITY OF HURRICANE CAMILLE OF 1969.

MOST OF THE AREA WILL BE UNINHABITABLE FOR WEEKS...PERHAPS LONGER. AT LEAST ONE HALF OF WELL CONSTRUCTED HOMES WILL HAVE ROOF AND WALL FAILURE. ALL GABLED ROOFS WILL FAIL...LEAVING THOSE HOMES SEVERELY DAMAGED OR DESTROYED.

THE MAJORITY OF INDUSTRIAL BUILDINGS WILL BECOME NON FUNCTIONAL. PARTIAL TO COMPLETE WALL AND ROOF FAILURE IS EXPECTED. ALL WOOD FRAMED LOW RISING APARTMENT BUILDINGS WILL BE DESTROYED. CONCRETE BLOCK LOW RISE APARTMENTS WILL SUSTAIN MAJOR DAMAGE...INCLUDING SOME WALL AND ROOF FAILURE.

HIGH RISE OFFICE AND APARTMENT BUILDINGS WILL SWAY DANGEROUSLY...A FEW TO THE POINT OF TOTAL COLLAPSE. ALL WINDOWS WILL BLOW OUT.

AIRBORNE DEBRIS WILL BE WIDESPREAD...AND MAY INCLUDE HEAVY ITEMS SUCH AS HOUSEHOLD APPLIANCES AND EVEN LIGHT VEHICLES. SPORT UTILITY VEHICLES AND LIGHT TRUCKS WILL BE MOVED. THE BLOWN DEBRIS WILL CREATE ADDITIONAL DESTRUCTION. PERSONS...PETS...AND LIVESTOCK EXPOSED TO THE WINDS WILL FACE CERTAIN DEATH IF STRUCK.

POWER OUTAGES WILL LAST FOR WEEKS...AS MOST POWER POLES WILL BE DOWN AND TRANSFORMERS DESTROYED. WATER SHORTAGES WILL MAKE HUMAN SUFFERING INCREDIBLE BY MODERN STANDARDS.

THE VAST MAJORITY OF NATIVE TREES WILL BE SNAPPED OR UPROOTED. ONLY THE HEARTIEST WILL REMAIN STANDING...BUT BE TOTALLY DEFOLIATED. FEW CROPS WILL REMAIN. LIVESTOCK LEFT EXPOSED TO THE WINDS WILL BE KILLED.

AN INLAND HURRICANE WIND WARNING IS ISSUED WHEN SUSTAINED WINDS NEAR HURRICANE FORCE... OR FREQUENT GUSTS AT OR ABOVE HURRICANE FORCE...ARE CERTAIN WITHIN THE NEXT 12 TO 24 HOURS.

ONCE TROPICAL STORM AND HURRICANE FORCE WINDS ONSET...DO NOT VENTURE OUTSIDE!

Because of Rick's bulletin, thousands of people safely evacuated as Hurricane Katrina approached the Gulf Coast. The catastrophic damage wrought upon New Orleans and the Mississippi coast proved Rick's bulletin tragically accurate, but even more would have died if not for his stark analysis.

Just as with an approaching storm, getting and embracing the right information when dealing with burnout is critical. If you don't know what's going on and don't have a plan, you're on dangerous ground. Having the right information, even if it's frightening to take in, allows you to formulate a solid plan.

Most people don't plan their lives. This lack of planning bites them when burnout hits. As development guru, Jim Rohn said, "If you don't plan your life, you'll fall into someone else's plan. And guess what they have planned for you? Not much!!" If you want to break out from burnout, start planning your life today.

People stuck in burnout don't plan ahead. Each day is a battle for survival in a high-pressure work environment or overstressed home front. Yet, the very act of setting goals and developing a plan to reach them is a key factor in overcoming burnout.

If you are stuck in burnout, today is the best time to develop a plan to get unstuck. The good plan you implement today is infinitely better than the perfect plan that you never actually execute.

On November 23, 1984, Boston College squared off against Miami in the Orange Bowl. Boston College trailed 45-41 with five seconds left in the game and the ball on the Miami 48-yard line. Boston College quarterback Doug Flutie dropped back to pass, evaded a sack, and tossed a 48-yard touchdown pass into the arms of receiver Gerald Phelan for the miracle win.

The pass, which became known as the Hail Flutie, helped Flutie win the Heisman at the end of the season. The Hail Flutie is a wordplay on the Hail Mary pass, a desperation pass typically thrown with time running out in an attempt for a miracle win.

Most Hail Mary's don't work, yet many people plan their lives with a Hail Mary approach. They start with noble intentions in the first quarter of their adult lives, with full intentions of winning at the game of life. They score some quick points by getting a degree, a spouse, some kids, and a mortgage. But life hits back hard, inflicting injuries and causing some fumbles. They stagger through the third quarter trailing, somehow trusting in a late-game miracle.

When burned out, you can feel like the coach trailing 34-6 with nine minutes to go in the game who continues to run the ball up the middle for short gains. Then, when it's too late, he starts airing it out and throwing long. When you're burned out, you can feel like a running back on that team trailing by four touchdowns in the fourth quarter, and the coach still tells you to run it up the middle on third and long.

Fortunately, life isn't a football game. Yet, people burning out often play the game of life like a quarterback with no authority to call a play. Who says you can't plan your own life? Who says you can't devise your own game plan? Who says you've got to pound it up the gut while getting your teeth knocked out by a bigger, stronger, faster opponent?

We've all heard the two-word phrase "they say". Who is "they"? "They" is whoever a burned-out soul allows to control them and call the shots. "They" can be a job that takes the best years of your life and gives you heartburn in return. "They" can be an unruly child who controls a parent through tantrums. "They" can be bureaucratic workplace devoid of common sense.

Burned-out people inevitably stop planning their lives and turn control over to the "they" voices in their life. "I'd have a wonderful life if THEY would let me." "I could achieve my dreams if THEY wouldn't get in my way." Frustration turns to anger because "they" provide the loud voice that calls the shots in a burned-out person's life. You cannot break out of burnout as long as others set your priorities.

So you wake up one morning and say, "I'M MAD AS (insert expletive of your choice) AND I'M NOT GOING TO TAKE IT ANYMORE!!" You march out and face life, complete with the friends, family, and coworkers who make up the "they" voices in your life. Tell them you've had it, and from now on you're calling the shots. Roll your eyes. Gesture with your hands. Let the whole world know just how serious you are about this. Then listen for their response. (Cue crickets chirping.)

Your family, friends, and coworkers have grown accustomed to you. Even if you've poured out your burnout frustrations to their sympathetic ears, your inner circle will often feel threatened by talk of change. The truth is most friends are not interested in your life plans. The same often holds for your family as well. They are interested in how you fit into their plans.

The same goes for institutions with which you may be

affiliated. Churches, professional associations, and organizations often work with the same goal in mind. They seek to get you involved in their activities. That's fine to a degree. Part of life is belonging to a community. Belonging to a community means joining said community in common activities. Your church seeks volunteers for keeping nursery, teaching classes, or singing in the choir. Your professional association requests your attendance at seminars and training programs. Your workplace requires your presence in job-oriented events.

Yet when dealing with burnout, an extra meeting here, a request to serve there, or "can we count on your attendance" elsewhere all adds up to living the agendas of others rather than your own. Organizations are staffed with positional leaders who measure success by how many people they can get involved doing their stuff. (A positional leader is someone who carries authority solely due to a position rather than influence.)

Positional leaders don't score points for helping you carry out your life plan. They get points in the eyes of their organization for getting you to do their stuff. Hence, the tug-of-war begins when a person who was only recently burned out, but compliant toward the wishes of others, begins to assert independence.

This is a tricky time in breaking out of burnout. We still have to do what the boss says at work. Unless we become a hermit, we still need to be involved with other people's interests. In the name of service, we still need to sometimes put aside our own selfish wants to help someone else. This means sometimes going along with that extra meeting called by a positional leader, even though you'd rather spend that two hours working your new life plan.

However, the road to burnout recovery contains an uphill grade of learning how to say no. Burned-out individuals have often become unwilling people pleasers who feel they must do whatever someone asks. Overcoming burnout means learning how to set your own agenda and secure some short-term wins doing your thing. As you build confidence in yourself, you can choose which outside activities warrant your involvement and which ones you should quit.

This is a particular challenge to burned-out folks with golden retriever personalities. Because of their general good nature, relational golden retriever types are often recruited to be part of someone else's team. That's because golden retrievers make excellent team members. However, while relational personality types make good team members, they often struggle when burned out to get other people interested in their plans. They can come to resent always being asked to sacrifice their own goals or plans for the plan of someone else.

Learn to listen to your own voice, develop your own life plan, and work that plan daily. No one else will work your plan for you. You possess sole responsibility for listening to the right voices and developing a plan for your life. However, when you begin formulating a plan for your personal development, keep one truth in mind.

Tip: Guard your dream, your time and your mind.

For starters, guard your dream. When you begin breaking out of burnout, you discover new passions and interests. Perhaps you rediscover a long-forgotten talent or hobby. You begin to dream about what to do with the rest of your life. Your natural tendency is to voice that dream to those around you. However, be careful with whom you share your dream.

Your dream may sound to a supervisor like a plan to change jobs. A know-it-all coworker may call your aspirations stupid. A cynical family member may dismiss your dream as yet another grand plan that will never happen. Others will try to shoot down your dream before it takes form. As motivational speaker Jeffrey Gitomer says, "People will rain on your parade because they have no parade of their own."

Should you zip your lip and keep silent? No. You need a few trustworthy friends who will encourage and hold you accountable. For example, when I decided to write this book, I told only a few people in my inner circle. My wife was a major source of support. I purposefully did not tell people who would not be enthusiastic about my journey.

When you burn out, those around you aren't exactly staring at the brightest bulb in the kitchen. Maybe they didn't always know to call it burnout, but they saw how you behaved. Perhaps you talked about big plans but never carried them out. Rather than giving others the power to cast doubt on your dream, start working to make it happen, and let them be impressed by the final result. They'll come on board soon enough when they see proof of positive change.

Secondly, guard your time. Statistically speaking, most millionaires in America are self-made. They weren't born rich. *The rich man and the poor man both have 24 hours in each day. The difference is how they spend their time.* Let that sink in for a minute. You can make things happen to get more money, but you can't get more time.

Burned-out people lose track of the weeks, the months, and too often the years. Time becomes a dreary clock on the wall, with eyes glued to the calendar waiting on Friday. When you binge-watch two 24-episode seasons of *Frankenstein Attacks Mayberry*, you can't get that time back. If you spend two hours a night watching the cable news, you can't get that time back. Life is too short to waste it listening to the voices of people shouting at each other.

This doesn't mean that we should never watch a goofy movie, a news talk show, or check Facebook. It means as you plan your life, you should also plan your day. I'll never be a happy to-do list-maker, but I've learned to prioritize the top two or three things that I absolutely need to do today, and do those things. If you are going to successfully break out of burnout, you'll have to master your schedule. Otherwise, you'll fall right back into "someone else's plan, and what do they have planned for you? Not much."

Finally, guard your mind. As you develop new priorities, hobbies, and a life plan, put the right things into your mind and keep the wrong things out. In burn-out mode, your idea of relaxing after a hard day might be to listen to Pink Floyd till 2:00 a.m. I've done that and thoroughly enjoyed it until I had to get up the next morning for work. However, now you need to reprogram your brain. This means listening to the right voices through books and teaching material. It could involve listening to motivational sermons and actually doing what the preacher says.

Tip: The biggest enemy in the war against burnout is the voice within your head.

As you break out from burnout, you will experience small but important victories, and start new habits that bring fresh energy. But you will inevitably have a bad day or a bad week. The car will have a flat, or a personal emergency will pop up, and the voice in your head will scream, "You can't do this. Your friend can but not you, because you're a loser." Guard your mind against negative ideas and voices.

Guard your mind against the wrong voices and tune your ear to the right ones. Just as Robert Ricks issued a bulletin of impending danger, keep your ears open to the right voices alerting you to danger in your fight to build a life of purpose. Don't listen to those who say "We've ridden the storm out before. We can stay put and come out alright." Not everyone survives the burnout wars with their dream and purpose intact. Supply yourself with the necessary tools to build a life of purpose.

    Why worry about the messaging in our head? Because soon after you burst forth to do battle with the forces of burnout, the forces of the cosmos will hit back with full fury to defeat your nascent journey into newfound freedom. You cannot escape this backlash. Like a hurricane heading directly at you, it will strike full force. You cannot avoid it. Accept that this counterattack will take place, and be ready to defeat it.

CHAPTER 10
PREPARE FOR THE BACKLASH

Burnout isn't going to let you go without a fight. As you begin your journey toward a new life, understand that a backlash is headed your way. How you handle this backlash will determine your level of success in victory over burnout.

Legions of people have started a worthy venture, only to quit when faced with this inevitable opposition that caught them unprepared or unwilling to fight back. The cosmos will not simply hand you the keys to your cell and bid you well as you walk out of burn-out prison. When you attempt to forge a new path, resistance to that effort is certain. The master jailer of burnout will not be happy with your decision.

Just as you think you've slipped away into a newfound freedom, rest assured the dragon of resistance will roar from its cave and seek to drag you, bound once again back to your prison. Just what is this demonic being that so fiercely strives to keep you from fulfilling your Divine destiny and living out the reason you were placed on this earth?

I sat at midfield in the Superdome, watching my team play in the Sugar Bowl. To the delight of the father in me, both my daughters marched in my alma mater's band at halftime. On this night, a life-dream came true, watching my own children play in the band, as my team won the Sugar Bowl. The game ended about 11:30 p.m. By the time we snapped selfies with the kids and exited the stadium, it was pushing midnight.

I will never forget the sight of thousands of football fanatics walking like a herd of cattle from the Superdome toward the New Orleans French Quarter. They strolled like zombies in a movie scene, mindlessly walking under the New Orleans street lights toward a land of bars with Hurricanes and Café Du Monde with beignets and café au lait.

As legions of hungry fans approached the French Quarter, an unfortunate thing happened. Most of the restaurants closed around midnight. After walking in this crowd of football zombies toward a perceived celebratory paradise, my family settled for pancakes at the only place in the exotic French Quarter we could find serving food, an International House of Pancakes.

This world is a funny place, in a pathetic sort of way. It proclaims to reward creativity and initiative. Yet, in reality, it offers the plain and ordinary. It promises New Orleans Cajun culinary delight and gives you ordinary pancakes. Filling, but mundane. In order to break out from burnout, you have to exert the extraordinary.

The cosmos exerts a subliminal force that causes us to walk in lockstep conformity. If you submit to this force, you are destined to a life as a "conformity zombie," wandering aimlessly through life, with the assurance you are traveling with the herd and the terror of not knowing where you are going. Conformity zombies demand that you go along with the crowd. They promise that in doing so you'll never be alone, yet they curse you to a life of wandering with no apparent direction. This is the epitome of burnout.

Our world insists on conformity. This insistence is natural to a degree, as the human race craves continuity in order to stay sane. Yet, this very conformity plays a major role in burnout. As humans, we possess wondrous, creative brainpower. When the cosmos insists on conformity, and we oblige out of peer pressure, it often cuts off the very creativity the world desperately needs from us. By conforming, we resign ourselves to a life of "what I could have been if only."

When breaking out of burnout, you will charge directly into the societal pressure to conform. Whether in the workplace or at home, the heavy boot of conformity presses hard upon your neck. When confronting the conformity zombies, do not despair. Just realize the battle has only just begun.

Burnout seems like a malady that all who care about you would want to see vanquished from your life. They would declare it to be true if asked. However, they don't think through the full ramifications of the effect your change will have on their life. Remember Newton's Law? *"An object at rest will tend to remain at rest until acted upon by an unbalanced force."* Even if others suspect you have a problem, they grow accustomed to you being at rest. You're a dependable lunch buddy.

You make them feel better about their life because they may be burned out too, and misery loves company. Your best friend at work may also be miserably burned out and look to you as a sympathetic shoulder upon which to cry. If you start getting better, it messes up your friend's comfort zone. The same scenario can play out with friends and casual acquaintances.

If your newfound independence means you now spend more time on personal development than on old activities, your old activity friends may feel abandoned. If in fighting burnout you decide to also lose weight and get in shape, you may come in conflict with friends accustomed to your old eating habits. Such people don't mean harm. However, your change affects their lives. Expect pressure to conform to old patterns, rejoin the old group, and order a thick and chewy pizza.

Tip: The conformity zombies don't want to kill you, but they will kill your dream by insisting that you put their priorities ahead of yours.

Just like the Sugar Bowl fans, they wander in the same general direction toward vibrant restaurants at closing time. You don't conquer burnout following the conformity zombies. A new hobby doesn't get explored, a second-income business doesn't get launched, or an online training course doesn't get completed by following the conformity zombies. Remember what zombies do. They try to turn you into a zombie as well.

Conformity has its place. You must conform to certain behaviors to function properly in society, to stay out of prison, and to keep your job. For purposes of overcoming burnout, pushing against conformity does not mean quitting your job as an Executive Vice President to become a free-love hippie. It means not letting outside forces derail your recovery by pressuring you to go back to your burnout mindset.

Just because you're breaking out of burnout, do not think for one minute that the surrounding system will applaud while you charge the horizon and boldly claim your creative spot. It will fight you, anonymous and nameless, like a horseman wearing a death mask. It dares you to charge and expects you to retreat in fear, yet it is willing to award victory to the brave soul daring to defy the odds and claim your mark that says, "I was here. My life mattered. I changed my little corner of the world."

Let's now assume that you get the memo and have squalled tires to escape the conformity zombies, safely heading to your new life, free of burnout and ready to reach your full potential. Just one more thing. The people around you insisting upon conformity are not the only enemies you face.

Just when you think you've got it together and turned life to the positive, you will come face to face with the biggest enemy of all. You can be on the moon, and this powerful nemesis will hunt you down. You might be one thousand miles from civilization in Siberia, and this beast-like creature can find you at midnight with no light. Who is this enemy? This real killer of hope?

Tip: Your biggest enemy is the person you see in the mirror.

An air of exhilaration strikes when you look into the rearview mirror and leave your burn-out days in the past. You start jogging before work and reading personal development books that tell you *how to kick burnout in three easy steps*. You're good! You're on your way to a new you! Then one day you stop at the signal light of life and wham! You get rear-ended. When you step out of your vehicle to identify the culprit, you look into the driver's seat in the car behind you only to see yourself!

You didn't get burned out by accident. Though you didn't realize it at first, your burnout came because, at some point in your past, you quit working on yourself. Little by little, you gave in to your lesser tendencies. Weaknesses overcame strengths. Fear replaced courage. Apathy replaced hope. Those weaknesses, fears, and apathetic attitudes were not instilled by others. They exist within you. They exist within us all, just waiting to strike.

This malicious force within seeks to kill us all, at least in terms of our ability to change. Call it the murderer of hopes and dreams. It will stop at nothing to sidetrack your life and all the good you now wish to accomplish. It is your most fearful enemy, and it is You. The most formidable force you encounter when breaking out of burnout is yourself.

Many of your friends will ultimately like the new you. They may be jealous at first because you're doing something positive and they are not, but they notice and may even be inspired by your efforts. The boss? Any boss with two brain cells to rub together wants a happier, more productive employee. The same principles that overcome burnout also work to improve your life in many other areas, including on the job productivity.

But deep within our human psyche lies fear. Fear of failure, fear of the unknown, fear of rejection. An old preacher once said "New levels, new devils." When you put basic improvement principles into practice, you overcome obstacles only to wake up and realize even more obstacles have now arisen. It's as if life says, "She handled that test okay. Now, let's see how she handles THIS!"

Nothing stays the same. When overcoming burnout, you don't return to your old world as a new and improved you. You return to a new world constantly adapting and changing, which presents new and more complex challenges. You get six months into a personal improvement regimen, then comes a bad news phone call out of the blue. A family member gets an ominous diagnosis. Financial troubles hit your workplace.

Be ready for the bomb to drop, because it will. When this bomb goes off in the middle of your new life, the enemy within cries out, "I knew this wouldn't work!" The old habit that you recently put down beckons. The new habit that transformed your daily routine gets shoved aside by the tyranny of the seemingly urgent. Suddenly, your dream crashes to the ground, shattering like glass into a thousand tiny slivers.

"No use, might as well give up, I'm just not meant to be a success," the enemy within wails. Yet, the enemy within has one great weakness. It has no will of its own. It can cry, scream, lie, and call you a loser. But it cannot force you to do its bidding. This enemy is part of you, but it does not have power over you. It is your dark side, your dark nature, and we all have it. We all have our inner Mr. Hyde that turns our best Dr. Jekyll from a respectable human being into a raving lunatic.

This enemy can call you a fat slob, but it cannot put a gun to your head and force you to eat a dozen jelly doughnuts rather than yogurt. It can call you a lazy procrastinator, but it cannot handcuff you and keep you from working an hour a day on a new endeavor. It can call you a stupid dummy, but it cannot block your entrance to an online classroom.

Anytime you try to better yourself, you meet the enemy within. This enemy will resist, protest, and throw tantrums. To truly breakout of burnout, you must learn to tune this inner demon out. Eat the yogurt, work an hour a day on the new venture, or take the online class.

Be ready for the fight. Be ready to resist the conformity zombies. Most of all, be ready for the battle within. To truly overcome burnout, this battle must be fought and won.

Now it's time to put your plan into action. This is where the fun begins. Burnout has been kicking your butt for a long time, but now you're going to kick back.

CHAPTER 11
TAKING ACTION

When breaking out of chronic burnout, there's nothing more exhilarating than taking action to reclaim your life. You are now at the point to start the journey toward personal reclamation. However, it's not enough to step out and start doing stuff. You must do the right stuff.

You may have heard how federal agents are taught to detect counterfeit money, not by spending time examining phony bills, but by studying the real thing carefully. Agents are taught the meticulous details of printed money, so when they encounter a fake, they know it. The same thing holds true in overcoming burnout. You don't study burnout itself. You intentionally study how to build a successful life.

Tip: You must be purposeful when overcoming burnout.

Things won't get better someday "just because." Recovery from burnout doesn't automatically happen. You don't pick it up by osmosis or just get over it. You must commit to doing the right things daily that bring growth to your life. Start with goal setting.

I have a friend who built a successful financial investment business. One day over lunch I asked, "How did you build your business?" He replied, "Baker, I set goals. I set daily goals, weekly goals, monthly goals, and yearly goals." He explained that, if he met his weekly goals, he rewarded himself by playing golf on Friday afternoons. Then came the kicker. "If I didn't make my weekly goals, I punished myself by staying in the office on Friday afternoon and making calls," he stated.

You won't get that little bit of advice from most self-help books. The very idea of punishing yourself for not meeting a weekly goal is anathema in today's modern society. However, my friend has succeeded financially because of radical attention to setting and achieving goals.

Tip: Winners set and achieve goals. Losers don't.

No one ever succeeded by accident. Success may have an element of being at the right place at the right time, but only if the individual is prepared. This comes by setting goals and working to achieve them. If you want to break out of burnout, get your hammer and chisel ready.

Goal setting must be joined by a commitment to personal growth. A person in burnout has stopped setting meaningful goals and isn't consistently working to improve. When burned out, you're often too busy jumping when someone else yells frog to spend time and effort on personal improvement.

Start by making two lists. The first is a six-month goals bucket list. This list can include places you want to go or things you want to do, provided they can be done within the next six months. You may want to save a thousand dollars for an emergency fund, run a 5k, or visit the mountains. Those things are reasonable within a six-month window. Put as much stuff on this list as you want, as long as you can do it within six months.

There's no magic in six months. You can do a three-month list or a one-year list. However, you want the time period to be short enough to reach the goal soon. Don't put going back to medical school or moving to a foreign country on this list. You want this list to be things that you can expect to accomplish in the near future.

Six months is long enough to accomplish a goal that stretches you just a bit. Attending the World Series in October can be on the list. Binge watching your favorite baseball team on television all summer should not. Pick some fun goals to make life interesting. A fishing trip to the mountains or that vacation you've been putting off because "they can't get along without you at work" could definitely make the list.

Put some things on the list that will stretch you. Training for a race, losing twenty pounds, or taking a night class could go on this list. The list should be a mix of fun and challenging goals. However, don't put more things on this list than you can accomplish in six months. That could lead to the abandonment of your goals.

When you've worked up a good list, tell someone you can trust. You need accountability in your new life, and this is a great place to start. I repeat, *tell someone you can trust.* If you're planning to hike Pikes Peak in three months, you don't need someone spouting "Why would you do something stupid like that?" Better yet, get a friend who will climb Pikes Peak with you. You'll have accountability and a training partner.

Local running clubs are great for this type of goal. Most have Couch to 5K programs packed with other beginners for friendship and accountability. Make the developing of new friends a key component of your breakout from burnout. Build fun into your list. Burnout is the pits, and now you need some good, positive enjoyment.

Now for the challenging part. Put a couple of things on your list that will cause you to grow personally. Perhaps you set a goal to spend a specific amount of time each morning for prayer and meditation. Spiritual vibrancy is a strong antidote to burnout. Read a book on a subject you enjoy that will expand your mind. I read *Gulag Archipelago* a few years ago. Author Aleksandr Solzhenitsyn's literary style and the book's length created a challenging read, but it opened my mind to a world I could not otherwise imagine.

Don't put long-shot goals on this list. It needs to be something you can achieve within a six-month window. Avoid general, lofty goals that, if not reached, can set you up for disappointment. Just because you've dreamed of canoeing down the Missouri River, doesn't mean you should quit your day job and tip your oars in the water tomorrow. Long-shot goals often get burnout victims in trouble. You start off with a grand goal that would challenge the strongest of souls to complete and wind up quitting in despair two weeks later.

Tip: Save the breaking of New Year's resolutions for January, not for goal setting time.

Make these goals specific rather than general. "I'm going to become a public speaker" is a wish, not a goal. "I'm going to join a weekly speaking club next Monday" is a goal. (Some goals can be both fun and challenging.) You set yourself up for failure if your goals are too general. As with the fun items, tell someone you can trust about these goals as well. Better yet, tell someone who can join you in the journey.

Book clubs, fitness clubs, bridge clubs, and prayer groups can create a sense of excitement when you join and start doing something positive for yourself. Some people say *I could never do THAAAAT*. True, and some people stay stuck all their lives too. You don't have to be that person.

Don't sweat the goals list, and feel free to add or subtract from it over time. As I tell my process-oriented beaver friends sometimes, rules are meant to serve people, not the other way around. This list is meant to serve you. Don't turn it into a taskmaster to which you must submit daily. If you don't enjoy running, don't sign up for a 5k. Do something else that you enjoy. If you don't like to read, find a growth activity that you enjoy and do it. It's a practical way to get moving forward and should bring value to your life in the process.

Now for the second list, your *growth* list. This list contains only two or three items at the beginning. While a goals list contains things you do, like a daily to-do list, a growth list involves key areas of life in which you seek to improve. Working on yourself is key to overcoming burnout. Remember, people in burnout have long since quit working on themselves. The purpose of setting some realistic, short-term goals is to get you doing something that you enjoy and will bring positive results to your life. This should give you some "quick wins." While vital, this is not the entire picture.

Start with two areas in which you wish to improve. One of these should be an area of strength. Choose something in an area of personal talent or giftedness and work each day to get better. Secondly, pick an area of choice in which you want to improve and spend time working on it each day. Dedicate 30 minutes daily to each area. Since you'll be working on these areas daily, your growth list should be short.

I once met a successful individual who was a college football All American in a top ten program years ago. He shared that his team didn't run a fancy offense. In fact, they ran only a handful of plays, but they drilled them over and over in practice until they ran them very well. Your growth list is your playbook. Make it short, with a couple of things that will rock your world by drilling these plays daily.

Your growth list contains two disciplines that you work 30 minutes *daily*, as in seven days a week. Don't let up because burnout is a deadly enemy that seeks to take you down. This growth list is your emotional and intellectual workout plan. If you go to the physical therapist with back pain, your therapist may give you a sheet diagrammed with exercises. You are told to repeat those exercises daily, *and, if you do them, you'll get better.* Same with your growth list. Except you get to choose what goes on this list.

Let's drill into what should go on this list. Your area of strength is something that you already do well. For example, you may have a knack for speaking before a crowd but haven't really honed the skill. You rely on your gift of gab for getting you through a presentation. However, if you spend 30 minutes a day, every day working on this gift, you could go from being a good talker to a great speaker. You may be a good short order cook in the kitchen. Thirty minutes a day studying your craft could make you a great chef, and bless those who eat your food in the process.

Tip: Don't put an area of weakness on this list as your "strength."

Don't spend a lot of time and effort on improving low-aptitude weaknesses. If you don't have a mechanical bone in your body, don't spend the bulk of your time studying auto-mechanics. If you hate math, don't go back to night school to study calculus.

Remember the 80-20 rule. Spend 80% of your time on the top 20% of your strengths and you'll get through the roof results. Conversely, spend only 20% of your time on areas of weakness. No one is the entire package. If you work hard to improve an area of weakness, you'll at best only become average in that area. If you work to improve a skill or strength, you can become great in that area. If you dedicate 30 minutes a day to a single strength, you can become an expert in that area within a year.

Also, choose a personal area in which you wish to grow. This could be your attitude, spiritual journey, or a field of study. If you would like to overcome shyness, spend 30 minutes a day intentionally greeting people in a friendly manner. You could spend 30 minutes a day reading in a subject pertaining to your profession and become well-versed in your field within a year.

Be purposeful about your growth, and tell your goals to an interested person who can hold you accountable. When you engage in personal growth and start achieving planned goals, burnout will lose its hold on your life. You simply can't be in positive growth mode and also be stuck in burnout.

When you're burned out, getting motivated to make positive changes can be difficult. When you've got the blues, it may seem perfectly normal to drown your sorrows in a bottle of Old Cadaver. All those pesky people out jogging appear as lunatics. You may wonder if the day will ever come when you feel energized again.

Don't wait on your feelings to change before tackling the burnout monster. You must act your way to a new way of thinking. Take the right actions, and the feelings to support these actions will follow. You may not arrive at your new destination overnight, but when you start planning your life through goal setting and personal growth, positive results will follow.

Now that you're on the road to setting goals and becoming a person who makes things happen, it's time to broaden your approach. To break out of burnout, you've got to get the right people in your life and the wrong people out of your life. While not always easy, it's a necessary step toward defeating chronic burnout.

Some people will offer encouragement and wise counsel along your journey. Others will douse you with gasoline and offer you a cigarette. So let's talk about how to get the first type of person in your life and the second type of person out of your life.

CHAPTER 12
MAKING THE RIGHT FRIENDS

Look at the people you hang around. In time, you will become who they are. If you hang out with winners, you will become a winner. If you hang out with morons, you will become a moron. Even if you've got a good brain upstairs, you will inevitably come to act like the people around you.

Burned out people tend to congregate with other burned out people. Understand right now that this dynamic must change and that you're the only one who can change it. If your best friends are coworkers with whom you complain about the job, what type of person do you start looking for when fighting burnout?

A few years ago, I was discussing by phone my goals with a life coach. Midway through the conversation, she asked me, "Where do you want to be in six months?" I thought for a moment and replied, "I don't know." She wouldn't let up and kept pressing me to think specifically about where I wanted to be in six months. Because of her insistence, I developed a six-month action plan that transformed my life. Without that question that day, I might have still been stuck six months later.

Motivational speaker Charlie Jones often said, "*You will be the same person in five years as you are today except for the people you meet and the books you read."* Let's consider the genius in that simple statement. In this chapter, we will look at the people you meet. Consider the five people in your closest inner circle. In five years, your life will resemble those five people.

If your foxhole buddies are vibrant and positive, you will become a vibrant, positive person. If your foxhole buddies are complainers, you'll become a complainer. A critical component of overcoming burnout is surrounding yourself with the right people.

By the time burnout hits, you've stopped working on yourself. Your priorities are primarily set by others, and you feel powerless to reverse this dynamic. You put others first and yourself last, but more from fear of peer disapproval than altruistic selflessness. This is a recipe for resentment and personal stagnation.

Tip: *Make meeting people who can positively impact your life a priority.*

Getting the right people to encourage your growth is crucial. Consider the people closest to you. Do they inspire you to become better? Are they positive role models? Have they accomplished a level of success in their personal or professional life that you have not? Do they encourage your efforts toward breaking out of burnout? If so, consider yourself fortunate.

However, what if the people closest to you do not inspire you to become better? What if they don't model success in their own lives? What if they have not accomplished success in areas where you need to improve? What if they discourage your efforts to overcome burnout? If so, you may need to get some new friends.

You have to do what it takes to bring the right people into your life and show the wrong people the door. Do not spend time with people who are not thrilled with your progress. If you become purposeful about growth, you'll outgrow many around you.

People with small dreams are content living their lives surrounded by other "small dreamers" who don't rock the boat. This does not make them unimportant. It does not mean they can't enjoy their work or have happy lives, good marriages, and loving children. It does mean they are content with mediocrity. Small dreamers don't often burnout in the sense of a mid-career stall.

Conversely, people who burn out tend to have large dreams. They harbor the belief that their lives should make a big difference in this world. They want to help people. When this belief is backed up by the ability to make a large dream come true, being surrounded by people who don't share those aspirations can kill dreams.

This dilemma exists for people who want to help others, want their lives to matter, yet find themselves stuck in jobs that have become all about the work. Does your inner circle of friends and co-workers encourage you to grow or to drown your sorrows with them down at the Dusty Mule?

Life is hard. It's a lot easier to throw in the towel and go along with the conformity zombies. If you want to break out of burnout, you've got to get busy developing new relationships with people who make you better. How do you find these beacons of positivity in a workplace full of Negative Nellies and a boss who's also burned out and hanging on for retirement? How do you find people who will ask you, "Where do you want to be in six months?" when the voices of your own family, friends, and coworkers, whose stability relies on you remaining where you are now, cry for your round-the-clock attention?

Tip: *If the cupboard is bare, look elsewhere for food or go hungry.*

I once worked with a quick-witted news videographer famous for asking people in a perfect monotone, "How did you get to be so good so quick?" We'd get a laugh, but that's actually a good approach when looking for people who can help you improve. Do this exercise. Think of people you know who launched a successful enterprise or who overcame odds to succeed in life. Without the wise-guy intentions of my news videographer friend, ask them, "Can we get together for lunch? I'd like to know how you built your business. I'd like to hear your story. Tell me how you got to be so good so quick."

Let's say you approach three successful people with this question. Two of them may say "I'll get back to you." But the third one may say, "Are you available next Wednesday?" Now, you're in business. Get a notepad and write out some questions ahead of time. When you meet for lunch, after an appropriate time for small talk, get out your pad and pen and start asking your questions. Write down the answers. You'll be amazed at how they open up and the wisdom they share.

We often assume successful people were born with a silver spoon in their mouth. However, most built their success from scratch and don't often get asked how they did it. Many will be flattered by the request and can offer life-transforming advice.

Remember this. Don't waste their time. If you get a lunch meeting with that business leader, don't spend the entire time talking about sports or politics. If you do so, you won't get a second meeting. They could be spending time with a sales client, but they chose to spend it with you. Make it count by showing up prepared.

Learn something about them. Check their Linkedin profile for a couple of professional facts or read an online article about their field to show you did your homework. Showing up prepared could land you a second lunch meeting to learn even more. Finally, don't be a sap. You invited them to lunch. Even if they are rich, offer to pick up the tab. To find these types of people, you have to network. Houses of worship, business groups, and civic organizations are good places to start. You may say, "Those church people are hypocrites! Those business folks are stuck up! Those civic groups are boring!" Do you want to overcome burnout or not? Remember the saying, *if you always do what you've always done, you'll always be what you've always been.*

I heard a sales coach once exhort his audience that when they feel down to "Get up, suit up, and show up!" Burnout can kill your desire to meet positive, successful people. But if you want to break out of burnout, you've got to change your burned-out ways. That means getting a couple of key mentors who can speak wisdom into your life.

Personal Example: This type of mentorship can take different forms. When the current president of my board of directors took office, we began meeting for breakfast on a weekly basis. He is a successful business person, a church leader, and well respected in the community. He models congenial and prompt communications and follow-up. Rather than lecture, he leads by example.

Our relationship is not one of "Oh Swami, how did you get to be so good so quick?" Rather, we meet and discuss ways to move our organization forward. In the process, I become a more effective director and a better person. The consistent communication keeps me accountable, and our brainstorming sessions, combined with input from our leadership team, create better thinking than one person could produce.

You can also be mentored by people you've never met or, in some cases, even by people who are no longer alive. This does not mean conjuring up the spirit of Andrew Carnegie through a séance. It means using the power of media by watching or listening to motivational or personal growth material and by reading their books.

Free online material is an internet search and a couple of mouse clicks away. A search for "personal growth material" will get you started. If you're on a budget, resources such as YouTube have plenty of free training material to get you started. Just get a pen and pad and start taking notes. Numerous leaders of the personal development community have free audio recordings available online. *(We'll include a training material resource guide at the end of the book.)*

My daddy drilled two things into my head. You get what you pay for, and it only costs a little more to go first class. Daddy didn't spend money frivolously, but when he did purchase an item, he bought something to last.

When breaking out of burnout, embrace the idea of investing in yourself. Investment means putting resources into something in order to receive a future return. Burnout produces a poverty of the mind mentality. But just as new relationships cost personal time and effort, don't wince at spending a bit of cash on your new direction.

My initial climb out of burnout began with $150 spent for a one month, four-session goals-setting workshop. I signed up for the workshop thinking I'd set a goal and achieve it by the end of the month. Turns out, that workshop spawned a journey of personal development that will hopefully continue my entire life. That $150 has paid for itself many times over by the process it unleashed in my life.

Not long after that workshop, I began watching free online personal development videos. I heard ideas about developing your human potential that you don't hear every day in church or the workplace. Through this journey, I learned the value of searching for direction on your own and not merely accepting society's dogma.

I later spent $300 on a CD set of teachings from numerous development leaders, who recorded a single weekend session. About once a year, I still listen through all twenty of those CDs to drink in the teachings, wisdom, and advice from those sage leaders. This taught me the value of repetitive learning. In school, we are taught to cram our heads full of knowledge for an exam, spit it out on some paper, then promptly forget that material, and move on to the next subject.

However, that approach doesn't work in life. The advertising "Rule of Seven" holds that a prospective customer has to see or hear something seven times before it sticks in the brain. In today's social media society, we are bombarded with so much information daily that we need to go over information numerous times not only to learn it but also to remember it down the road.

Don't overlook live seminars that offer personal development, leadership, and growth training. These seminars can range from a $150 half-day session at the local community college to expensive week-long conferences that mix motivational training with practical tools designed to build value into your life. Choose the venue that best suits your moment in time.

Nationally known speakers and authors who have built successful enterprises know something that you and I don't. We can learn from their expertise by watching videos and attending conferences. Spend some time online watching the free material. Choose mentors who speak your language, and learn from them.

This part of the journey takes time. It takes hours to listen to a twenty CD set. A half-day seminar or two-day conference costs time and money. It's possible to overcome burnout without going to training conferences. However, keep your mind open to the possibilities of bringing the right people into your life through these methods.

It's critical to get the right people into your life, who encourage your personal development. You won't win the race running with the slow dogs. Start the process now of recruiting new people who will help you grow.

As you start working on meeting the right people, start reading the right books. I've learned that books unlock the key to wisdom. Wisdom unlocks the mind to possibilities never before imagined. Books teach you how to achieve those possibilities.

Breaking out of burnout comes with a price tag. For one, it will cost you some time and money creating your own personal library. Become a reader because *you will be the same person in five years you are today except for the people you meet and the books you read.*

CHAPTER 13
THE BOOKS YOU READ

Burnout happens because you run out of fuel. One of the best ways to refuel your mind is to read books that motivate and provide the tools to fight back and change your life. The information in good books, properly applied, can transform your life.

When my father passed away in 2004, I was married with two children, a 30-year mortgage, and no savings. His passing served as a wake-up call. Daddy left this world with no house note and a comfortable middle-class nest egg built on his wages as a sewing machine mechanic in a garment factory and my mother's salary as a school teacher.

With Daddy's example fresh in my mind, I read Dave Ramsey's *Total Money Makeover* and began applying those principles to my family finances. My wife and I started a rainy-day fund savings account. We upsized from our cramped starter home to a larger home with a 15-year mortgage. Today our home is paid off, and we have no debt. We did this on my salary as a homeless shelter director and my wife's pharmacist salary. The ideas applied from one book that cost $24.99 revolutionized our personal finances.

Books contain ideas, knowledge, insight, and inspiration. If you want to improve your life, become a reader. I've heard the saying that "Not all readers lead, but all leaders read." Studies show that financially successful people read daily to keep up with professional trends and ideas. While this is not a book on financial literacy, it's worth noting that reading ranks high on the priority list of successful individuals.

The burned-out mind is like a dry, used sponge that has become stiff over time. Stuck in the cabinet under the sink, this sponge looks pathetic until soaked in water. Likewise, a burned-out mind becomes dry and stiff without the water of new ideas. Just as applying water to a stiff, dry sponge makes it usable again, ideas bring new life and application to a dry, stiff brain.

When breaking out of burnout, books open our minds to a bigger world. They get us out of ourselves and highlight new possibilities and ways of thinking. Today you can download a Kindle book, and start reading within minutes. I'm old school and prefer a hard copy book to highlight, underline, and dog-ear. I like to make notes in the margins, complete with exclamation points and smiley faces when discovering an idea or quote that catches my attention.

Like anything worthwhile, reading takes time and focus. Before you say, "I don't have time to read," think about this. You will spend 24 hours each day doing something. It's one thing if you don't have time to read because you're currently launching a new project or working overtime as an accountant during tax season. It's another thing if you claim to have no time to read, yet make time to watch reruns of your favorite television shows each night.

Tip: Read books that teach what you need to know.

I spend a significant portion of my workweek in routine meetings, returning phone calls, and answering emails. I learned to chalk this up to serving as the director of an organization by reading *The Effective Executive* by Peter Drucker. This doesn't mean I have to like meetings, but it means, as an Executive Director, attending them goes with the territory.

I learned to focus your best talents on areas of opportunity rather than areas of need by reading *I'm a Lucky Guy* by Joseph Cullman, longtime Chairman of Phillip Morris. Burnout often causes people to exhaust energy working to meet the perceived needs of others. In overcoming burnout, learn to apply your talents long-term to areas of untapped opportunity.

By reading the Bible, I learned to understand the heart and mind of God. Its words have provided personal solace in times of loss and the comfort of knowing I'm not on this Earth by accident. I learned the power of building a team rather than going it alone by reading *The 21 Irrefutable Laws of Leadership* by John Maxwell. No one person is the total package. Therefore, it's critical to surround myself with people who are strong in areas of my personal weaknesses.

I learned the necessity of doing the hard work of summer to reap a harvest in the fall by reading *Philosophies for Successful Living* by Jim Rohn. Too many people want the big payday without hard work. When the initial excitement of spring gives way to the heat of summer, you must embrace the work of overcoming burnout.

You don't always know on the front end which books to read. My upstairs man-cave is filled with books of various types, some of which I've read cover to cover, others which I've partially read, and some I'll never read because they don't light my mental fire. Understand that you have to buy the book to read the contents. Some books will be a home-run and others a strikeout. Celebrate the home-run books, and don't sweat the strikeouts.

Read books that inspire. I learned the power of turning defeat into victory by reading Winston Churchill's *History of the Second World War.* Shortly after leading England to victory in World War II, Churchill was voted out of office as Prime Minister. Instead of whiling away the time in anger, he spent the following years composing his six-volume classic masterpiece.

Steven Pressfield taught me the value of savage allegiance to finishing a project in *Do the Work*. A college friend turned contemporary professor and author, Ellen Meacham, inspired me to write when I read her well-written and documented book titled *Delta Epiphany: Robert F. Kennedy in Mississippi*.

Read books that make you laugh. Burnout is not funny. It's hard to laugh when you've lost the energy to enjoy life. Books can both inform and entertain. Bart Yasso, the Chief Running Officer for *Runner's World*, brings running home in his book *My Life On the Run* through hilarious accounts of encountering rhinoceroses during a race, running the Antarctica Marathon, and his au naturale appearance in the textile-free Bare Buns Run. I keep Gary Larson's *Far Side* book in my office. On the most serious days, I often sneak a peek at the cartoon of a cat sharpening its claws on the wooden leg of an old sea captain.

What about alternative forms of learning? Not everyone is an avid reader. Some people prefer webinars or by watching how-to training videos. Some prefer to listen to audio books while traveling. Zig Ziglar often talked about "Automobile University" to describe the learning that takes place while listening to recorded audio teachings in your automobile. Some technology-oriented people prefer a Kindle e-book over paper. Some books are available for free online as a .pdf file.

You don't have to join a Book of the Month club to overcome burnout. I prefer a real book made from trees. Reading an internet article about Herman Melville will give you information about the famous author. Reading *Moby*

Dick will take you inside his soul. However, the internet has opened up new online opportunities for learning that can transform your mind.

Just realize that outside of the new people you meet, the new information you put into your brain will be a deciding factor in determining who you become. Just as with the question "Where do you want to be in six months?", ask yourself "Who do I want to be in six months?" Then read books to help you become that person you wish to be.

It's your decision whether you read and learn. The world is fine with you staying dumb. Just know this. The book you don't read can't inspire you. The book you don't read can't teach you what you need to know. The book you don't read won't make you laugh. The book you don't read can't illuminate new worlds in your mind. A person who doesn't read doesn't learn. If you choose to travel life without learning, you're like the person wearing a t-shirt that says on the back "I hate reading" and on the front "I'm with stupid" and an arrow pointing to your head.

Consider launching a post-burnout reading tour. I've shared with you some of the books from my tour. You should come up with your own books. How do you find them? An internet word search is a good place to start. Most books are purchased online today. Read the reviews and get started. Another place is a local bookstore. While not as common as in the past, most metropolitan areas still have a bookstore or two. If you become a reader of books on personal growth, you'll develop your favorite authors.

A word of caution on books. They are the source of life-changing ideas, *but only if you do the work of implementing the ideas in the books.* Some people become personal development junkies, reading their favorite authors and hopping from seminar to seminar with no genuine life change. They have little else than a hobby because they never take the step of translating the teachings into action.

Develop a "breaking out of burnout" library. Commit yourself to read a chapter a day of material that will help you grow. Start somewhere. Of all the things you do to overcome burnout, nothing has the potential to open your mind to new worlds and potential like the power of books.

Develop your own little book of quotes. When you come across a sentence or phrase that speaks to you, write it on an index card, including the author, book and page number. File it where you can find it. Later on, you'll have a system for finding the quote. You may prefer to keep notes on your phone, tablet, or computer. Find a method that works for you and do it.

A note about books. They can change your life. However, resist the temptation to tell dumb friends about the great book you're reading. That's because your friends don't care, particularly early on in your journey. Give the ideas you read time to bring about a visible change in your life. Wait for someone to say, "You've changed for the better. What did you do?" Then mention the book you read and how its ideas changed your life when you put them into practice.

When you read a book that rings your bell, read it again six months to a year later. The same layered learning that takes place when listening to the audio teachings applies for books. I read John Maxwell's *21 Irrefutable Laws of Leadership* and *Good to Great* by Jim Collins about once a year.

It's easy to read a book that opens your mind, then put it on the shelf and go your merry way thinking "Wow, that was such a great book. It changed my life!" A month later, if someone asks you about the book's contents, you look dumbfounded because you can't remember. I've read a book for a second time and thought, "This is good stuff. But I don't remember it from before." Because of that, I read some books more than once.

A note for avid readers. Consider taking a speed-reading course. You don't have time to read all the good books in the world. By speed reading, you learn to scan a book to see if it's worth your time for a more thorough read. Not all books are created equal, so don't waste time reading books that don't add value to your life. Yet, dedicate time each day to read books that help you grow.

Good books are like good friends. They are always there for you. They're like the friend you can go a decade without seeing, but, when you finally get back together, it's like you haven't missed a beat. Books are great educators. Because of Andrew Roberts' *Storm of War*, I'm a shade-tree expert on the epic World War II Battle of Stalingrad. It's doubtful I will ever travel to that corner of the world, but I've already been there in my mind. Develop an innate curiosity about life. Be the person who looks at the shelf in a bookstore and says "So many books. So little time!"

Make reading a new habit in your life. Most burned-out people have developed poor habits over time. You can't escape burnout by practicing the same old negative habits. Now that you're armed with the challenge to meet the right people and read the right books, it's time to get busy developing the right habits to break out of burnout.

CHAPTER 14
BREAKOUT HABITS

It's easy to develop a bad habit. Without much work, we can become an expert at a nagging tendency that creates problems. It won't be long before that bad habit produces some really rotten consequences. Running late to work, lack of personal growth, and sub-par performances are a few results from certain bad habits.

It takes hard work to develop good habits. Positive, productive habits don't happen naturally. However, good habits lead to higher productivity, including small things like showing up to work a few minutes early and meeting deadlines with time to spare.

A coffee mug recently caught my attention. In bold letters, the mug read "**I hate morning people. I hate morning. I hate people.**" As a night owl trapped in a morning lark world, this mug spoke to me. Morning people bounce out of bed at zero-dark-thirty, rush into work full of energy, and write the work schedules. Most night owls could qualify for a Nascar pole position driving to work because we hit the snooze button 28 times before slithering out of bed.

I joined a health club a few years ago and noticed workout classes scheduled for 5:30 a.m. In my view of the world, that's just sick. Yet, I needed a change in my morning routine and made the radical decision to attend the 5:30 a.m. workout classes for one week. I now get up at 5:00 a.m., go for a workout and emerge energized and ready to face the day. I initially thought my early morning workout would get my exercise done for the day. In the process, I discovered a *breakout habit*.

Tip: A breakout habit is one of the best weapons against burnout.

These are positive daily habits that launch a breakout effect in other areas of your life. I began attending the early morning workout classes to get in shape after a period of inactivity. However, working out in the early morning triggered unexpected but positive benefits beyond fitness.

I soon made friends in our classes who would ask "Where you been?" if I missed a class. This taught me accountability. It forced me to go to bed by 10:00 p.m. rather than staying up past midnight. After showering and getting dressed at the club, I was at work by 7:15 a.m., wide awake with my morning coffee and ready to face the day. While difficult at first, this routine became a habit.

Breakout habits trigger a series of benefits. Some good habits are singular in nature. But a breakout habit positively affects other areas of life, just as the first domino that gets tipped over causes the remaining dominoes in the line to tumble as well.

A habit initially meant just to address fitness triggered a breakout in the area of time management. I started getting up early, getting good exercise, prioritizing my daily goals, going to bed at a decent hour, losing weight, and becoming part of a new community. A habit started to get in better shape lead not only to better health but also to a better sense of well-being. Developing this single habit also taught lessons about disciplines and habits.

Developing positive daily habits is critical to overcoming burnout. People in burnout often develop bad coping habits and forego the practice of good habits. A burned-out mom too tired to cook after getting kids up for school and working all day may rely on fast food to feed herself and the family. A burned-out medical worker may forego exercise. A burned-out minister who would never drink or use drugs may overeat and become overweight. A burned-out counselor who doesn't identify as an alcoholic may knock the stress with a couple of drinks at night.

Over time, the fast food turns into a chronic unhealthy diet. Lack of exercise leads to extra pounds and a weaker heart. Overeating leads to diabetes and high blood pressure. A couple of drinks turns into alcohol dependence.

A breakout habit is an antidote to a burn-out induced slide into unhealthy living. Not everyone struggles in the same area, so there's no "one size fits all" breakout habit. Examine your life. What areas do you need to address? Ask yourself this question: *What is the one thing I can change today that would transform my life?* Develop a breakout habit around that one thing. Sometimes the "one thing" is stopping a destructive habit playing into your burnout. Therefore, a breakout habit could be a new routine to help overcome or replace a bad habit. Most burned out people have developed some bad habits they need to overcome.

In an earlier chapter, we discussed goals and goal setting. Goal setting and developing new habits are complimentary but not the same thing. Running the Slowpoke 5k is a goal. Jogging 30 minutes a day is a habit that helps you reach your goal. Losing 30 pounds is a goal. Eating a fruit and vegetable-based diet is a habit that helps you reach your goal. Getting in shape is a goal. Going to a workout class each day is a habit that helps you reach your goal. Gaining knowledge about personal development is a goal. Reading 30 minutes a day on the subject is a habit that helps you reach your goal.

Now we come to a difficult word. This word conjures up visions of stern taskmasters, drill sergeants, or staid librarians continually shushing you when you try to whisper. This word is d....di.....(dang, it's hard to say)....dis.....discipline!! There, I've said it. *The discipline of developing good habits is the difference between people who want to break out of burnout and those who actually do.* Many people know they are burned out but don't do anything about it because they lack discipline. If you want to break down the barn doors to burnout and ride into the pasture of a new life, it will take discipline. There's no way around it.

When you initially break out of burnout, you'll hit an emotional high. You read a book, hear a talk, listen to a sermon, and bounce forward feeling renewed and refreshed. For a few weeks, you hop out of bed with pep in your steps. You've left the prison cell called burnout behind, never to return. You may even declare that your burned out days are over. You're free!!

Then, *bam!!* Reality kicks you like a Missouri mule right between the eyes. A month after starting the early morning workout class, you come down with a sinus infection. You lose some weight on the new diet and then comes the family beach vacation and streets lined with seafood restaurants. You apply yourself to a daily regimen of renewal, reading, and meditation only to get an emergency call concerning a family member.

Suddenly, your best-laid plans are put on hold out of necessity. You can't work-out when running a fever. Can't diet on vacation. Can't spend time on personal renewal when you're in the emergency room with a family member. *When fighting your way out of burnout, rest assured a bomb will drop just when you think you're in the clear.*

When this bomb drops, you may fall back into old behaviors. This just means your human. Don't sweat gaining a few pounds on vacation. You can resume working out when the infection clears up. The family member will return home from the emergency room.

When life kicks you between the teeth and knocks you off your "breakout habit" game, pick yourself up, dust yourself off, and get back in the game. When your head clears, stick that CD back in the player, or fire up that motivational podcast. Return to the gym, or hit the walking trail. Get back on the diet, and start meditating and reading. Part of the discipline of burnout recovery is learning how to get back up when you fall.

The habit of bouncing back. Bonnie St. John had a leg amputated as a child. However, she fought back to compete in the 1984 Winter Paralympics in Innsbruck, Austria. St. John won a silver medal that year. On one particular race, she fell at a tricky spot on the course. She later said the person who won gold "also fell in that same spot. But she got up quicker. I learned that everybody falls down. Winners get up, and gold medal winners just get up quicker."

As you establish new habits to overcome burnout, you'll fall down sometimes. Your destiny depends upon how you respond. Oprah Winfrey was demoted on her first job as a TV anchor. The station didn't want to pay out her contract, so they demoted to her to host a talk show. Walt Disney was fired as a newspaper cartoonist in 1919 for "not being creative enough." One of Beethoven's early teachers said: "As a composer, he is hopeless."

When establishing new habits, resist the urge to move too fast. A wise preacher once said, "It's not how many miles you run in a day but how many days you run a mile." Defeating burnout is dependent on your steadfast daily work. The little disciplines you perform daily will lead to success.

If you are burned out, ask yourself, "How bad do I want to break out of this burnout?" It's possible to know you're burned out but not be willing to pay the price to overcome. I once worked with an alcoholic ex-offender, who had spent years in prison for small-time crimes. He left our rehabilitation program after being sober more than a year. Shortly after that, he was arrested for a small-time burglary. Sadly, prison was the life he knew and the place he felt comfortable. He committed a small felony because he would rather exist in prison than live free.

Why are habits vital to overcoming burnout? Because our habits define our destiny. The following quote has been attributed to numerous writers over the years. Those among us who would dare to attempt a noble life of purpose should heed it still today.

> *Sow a thought, reap an action.*
> *Sow an action, reap a habit.*
> *Sow a habit, reap a character.*
> *Sow a character, reap a destiny.*

Your habits will define you. They will shape you. They will make or break you. Establish good habits. However, do not think that reading a compelling quote is enough to get you on the right road. If you're burned out in mid-life, establishing positive new habits can be a life-transforming experience. However, it will not be an easy venture, especially when combating the darker side of your own nature. While worthwhile, it is never easy.

- Gaining weight-easy.   Losing weight-hard.
- Beer gut-easy.   Six-pack abs-hard.
- Watching late night tv-easy. Taking a night class-hard.
- Checking social media-easy.   Taking an online class-hard.
- Dropping out of school-easy. Getting your G.E.D. later in life-hard.

Life is full of easy roads to nowhere. However, the road to success is paved with discipline and hard work. Discipline is not some amorphous, existential concept. It is a concrete reality that you must practice each day. You can read volumes on discipline, but, until you start practicing a discipline daily, it will not do you one bit of good. No good discipline is too small to grant some benefit. No bad habit is too small to cause some harm. The greater the discipline, the greater the benefit. The greater the bad habit, the greater the harm.

If you desire to overcome burnout, define a breakout habit that, when triggered, will transform your life. Then begin working that habit with discipline each day. Be ready to fight, because your dark side and weaknesses will push back against these new habits.

A personal note. Some disciplines may cause a positive change in behavior but will not change your personality. I am a night owl by nature. I have modified my behavior in a positive way that allows me to function with energy in the morning. Being a night owl is not a character defect. It does not define success or failure. I simply work in a world where staying up until 2:00 a.m. and sleeping till 10:00 a.m. does not work.

Therefore, I developed a breakout habit to help deal with that situation. However, I sometimes allow myself the luxury of staying up late on Friday night and sleeping in on Saturday mornings. So, depending on the habit, allow yourself room to be human. Some people advocate working on your new habits daily no matter the situation. Others allow an occasional cheat day. Find and practice what works for you.

Your breakout roadmap may consist of goals and growth initiatives. However, the engine of your breakout will be powered by discipline. You cannot avoid it. Start working on good daily habits today.

You won't develop good habits by accident. You've got to have a plan. A "good habits" plan is different from a goal setting plan. This action plan is where meeting the right people, reading the right books, and developing good habits moves from the realm of good ideas to action.

You can read this book and think it's swell. However, if you don't develop and implement an action plan, you'll stay stuck in burnout. You've come this far, so let's get busy putting your plan together.

CHAPTER 15
ACTION PLAN

Merriam-Webster defines a plan as *a method for achieving an end*. Whether you succeed at breaking out of burnout depends solely on your willingness to develop and implement a method to do that very thing. It won't happen any other way.

When my first daughter was born, my wife and I didn't know what to do. The little bundle of joy came into the world screaming and, even as an adult, she hasn't shut up. During those first nights of 2:00 a.m. feedings, diaper changes, and a baby who wouldn't quit screaming, I didn't feel this automatic flow of fatherly love. I didn't even know this thing that had invaded my predictable world. She didn't come with a "how to" manual.

However, I soon fell in love with this baby and have had the privilege of watching her grow up into a beautiful, intelligent, and vivacious young woman. As you struggle through the early stages of breaking out of burnout, a similar journey lies ahead. At first, you wrestle with the emotions of planting the seeds of a new tomorrow and plucking out some old stuff that holds you back.

You realize the need to break down old obstacles, and build new roads of habits and thought patterns that move you to a new place in life. Some days you will struggle with the weirdness of a new habit foreign to your old self. In time, you will come to know and love the new direction, new people, and new vigor that a life free of burnout holds.

Tip: To make this happen you have to get started.

Get started by working an action plan. Don't wait until you have everything worked out perfectly. As General George Patton said, "A good plan today is better than a perfect plan next week." While I cannot lay out your plan for you, here are some suggestions.

Get the right information. Purchasing and reading your first personal development book is a good start. ***We include a resource guide at the end of this book with suggestions to get you started.*** I recommend a real book with paper that you can own, write your name in, and mark it however you like. If you prefer a tablet, many of those also allow for underlining. The key is getting the right voices speaking into your head. It's also important to tune out the wrong voices. You must decide whether to listen to positive voices steering you forward or negative voices saying don't change.

Begin establishing a new breakout habit now. Starting a breakout habit provides evidence of real, tangible progress. It changes your routine and provides the momentum of moving forward. It's like taking a cruise. You plan, pack, arrive at the port of embarkation, and board the ship. But when those big engines start vibrating and the ship starts moving, you get a tingle of excitement knowing that your cruise is actually underway. Starting a new habit signals your brain and body that your voyage away from burnout is underway.

Start practicing a hobby. Dust off an old interest, or take up something new. If you're dealing with workplace burnout, it's not always possible or advisable to switch jobs. However, a new hobby gives you something new and interesting to think about and do. *It's important to not just have a hobby, but to practice the hobby.* If you enjoy playing guitar but haven't strummed your six-string since Old Buck was a calf, you only have an interest. Practicing the guitar 30 minutes a day is a hobby. Always wanted to take guitar lessons? Jump in and start!

Make a new friend. Or two. It can be someone you meet at the fitness club, a civic club, or at church. It's important to make a new friend outside your current friendship loop to share your new breakout journey. Old friends often don't understand your desire to change and may even have a vested interest in you staying the same. For example, if you want to join a speaker's club as a hobby, make a new friend at the club who shares your interest in speaking.

Start a personal development notebook, and write out a plan. A regular three-ring notebook will do fine. Write out your commitment to new habits. List the habits you wish to develop. Set some realistic goals and write them out. *Then share your plan with another trusted person.*

Tip: There's an old saying that "In business, nothing happens until something gets sold." In breaking out of burnout, nothing happens until you take action.

However, when you take those first steps, something exhilarating happens. Your coworkers may not understand. Your spouse, kids, or parents may not get it. Yet, you know that, in order to be true to yourself, you have to start something new. When you actually break the first piece of ground, the feeling of working toward a harvest keeps you going.

When I was a kid, I remember when my daddy decided to plant a garden. We planted good stuff like corn, peas, squash, green beans, and okra. However, radishes were the first edible item the garden produced. I don't particularly like radishes, but the excitement from eating something we grew by the sweat of our brow on our land was enough to make me wolf down those radishes.

In your breakout plan, plant some proverbial radishes. While your long-term goal consists of peas and okra, the radishes will provide the excitement of a quick win. Your long-term goal may be a career change or a job move. The six-month goal achievement of completing an online training course or finishing the Over the River Run gives the sense of accomplishment that lets you know greater things await. Embrace the small victories.

CHAPTER 16

CONCLUSION

Now for some tips, pointers and random closing thoughts.

- You now have a "no excuses" life in front of you. Don't wait for the perfect time to make changes because the perfect time will never arrive.
- Put yourself first, not out of selfish motives, but because you cannot give to others what you do not have. You cannot grow except by working on yourself. This means at least for a couple of hours each day, put yourself first.
- Don't neglect your spiritual development. You will not defeat the demons in your life through anger, envy, jealousy, and resentment. Many people attack religion today, but a good religion always encourages us to be our best. The world needs your best.
- Don't be a complainer. Nobody likes being around a chronic whiner. The sooner you begin working to improve your life rather than complaining, the happier you'll be. I've never seen a person who is both angry and happy at the same time.
- Attract your own luck. The saying goes that luck happens when "preparation meets opportunity." If you do the work of personal preparation, "good luck" will follow in time.

- Realize this journey will not turn out as you planned. You can draw up a great plan with awesome goals only to have the opportunity to turn up under some rock you never imagined.
- Become a person of discipline. Out of shape slobs don't win the Olympics.
- When you're at work, work. When you're at play, play. Even if you have the worst job ever, give it your best. The discipline will carry over. When spending time with the kids, forget about work for a minute.
- Don't try to maintain the status quo. Change the status quo by changing what you do each day.
- Don't spend time with people who aren't excited about your personal growth.
- Don't wait for others to make you happy. Create your own happiness.
- Don't take your dreams to the grave. Live them out while you still draw breath.
- Go see your favorite band in concert while you still can.
- You only get one life. Live it to the fullest.

Life contains precious few guarantees. You can follow the recommendations in this book and still get struck by lightning. However, I can promise that, if you are burned out, you can develop a plan to break out of burnout, and have a wild ride in the process.

Ask yourself "What type of person do I want to be? One who makes it happen, watches it happen, or wonders what happened?" A person who wonders what happened probably isn't reading this book. A person who makes it happen might be too busy making it happen to read this book.

That leaves the "watch it happen" group. If you have watched it happen until now, but desire to make it happen in your life, take heart. Wishing and hoping won't make it happen. However, if you are willing to develop a plan to improve your life and act on your plan, sparks will fly.

Know that if you consistently work the process, you will launch an exciting, bumpy, uneven, unpredictable breakout of burnout. In doing so, you just may discover your ultimate purpose for being on this earth.

When you complete the book, please leave an honest review on Amazon!

If you are burned out and seek to regain control of your life, download my free resource and start the journey of rebuilding your life today.

4 Steps to Taking Back Your Life by Taking Back Your Day

https://rexbaker.ck.page/95c215070d

A Suggested Resource List

"Philosophy for Successful Living" by Jim Rohn. (Easy read packed with life-changing advice.)

"Change or Die" by Alan Deutschman. (Outlines how radical change is more transforming than incremental change.)

"Managing Oneself" by Peter F. Drucker. (Classic, easy read by the leader in personal and corporate management.)

"The Strangest Secret" by Earl Nightingale. (Best-selling audio recording from the 1950s on the secret to success. Available online.)

"The 15 Invaluable Laws of Growth" by John C. Maxwell. (Practical treatise on the process of personal development.)

"Jim Rohn Complete Guides Set" by Jim Rohn. (A quick reading 5 booklet set that will change your life if you do what it says for the cost of about $15.00)

"Rich Habits" by Tom Corley. (Short, thought-provoking book comparing the daily habits of rich people and poor people.)

"The Richest Man in Babylon" by George Clason. (Easy reading book with sage advice for financial and life planning.)

"The Power of Habit" by Charles Duhigg. (In-depth book detailing the power of habit in our lives.)

"Good to Great" by Jim Collins. (Classic read demonstrating what successful organizations do and what unsuccessful organizations do not do.)

"The One Thing: The Surprisingly Simple Truth Behind Extraordinary Results" by Gary Keller and Jay Papasan. (Inspiring book on prioritizing your most important goal and the time-management necessary to make it happen.)

Made in the USA
Coppell, TX
09 September 2020

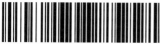